"Keith McCormick is a brilliant, courageous pioneer who, in this long-awaited guide, has torn away the curtain from the mystery of osteoporosis. Anyone seeking to renew their bone health will find the information presented in this meticulously researched handbook totally accessible, eminently usable, inspiring, and life-changing. This is a seminal work that will transform the way osteoporosis is treated in this country and will be referenced for years to come both by physicians and the general public."

> —Richard L. Gerstein, MD, chief medical officer at Baystate
> Mary Lane Hospital in Ware, MA

"To build better bones, you'll need to do way more than pop calcium pills and take walks. Now you can get inside information from the bone health guru. If you are planning on living a long life, you will need great bones. Don't hesitate—grab this book and take action!"

> —JJ Virgin, Ph.D., CNS, CHFI, nutritionist, fitness expert,
> and author of *The Art of Losing It*

"A savvy and practical self-help approach to osteoporosis. This necessary manual is crafted by a healer keenly attuned to the subtle interdependencies between bone health and exuberant, whole-body health."

> —David Abram, author of *The Spell of the Sensuous*

"Who would have thought that a reference guide on the prevention, diagnosis, and treatment of osteoporosis could be such a page-turner? This delightful gem of a book is truly a masterfully crafted, informative, and deeply satisfying read. It is most certainly destined to become a classic in the field of bone health."

> —Martha Stark, MD, clinical instructor in psychiatry at Harvard
> Medical School

THE WHOLE-BODY APPROACH TO OSTEOPOROSIS

HOW TO IMPROVE BONE STRENGTH AND REDUCE YOUR FRACTURE RISK

R. KEITH MCCORMICK, DC

NEW HARBINGER PUBLICATIONS, INC.

Publisher's Note

This publication is designed to provide accurate and authoritative information in regard to the subject matter covered. It is sold with the understanding that the publisher is not engaged in rendering medical, psychological, financial, legal, or other professional services. If expert assistance or counseling is needed, the services of a competent professional should be sought.

Care has been taken to confirm the accuracy of the information presented and to describe generally accepted practices. However, the authors, editors, and publisher are not responsible for errors or omissions or for any consequences from application of the information in this book and make no warranty, express or implied, with respect to the contents of the publication.

The author, editors, and publisher have exerted every effort to ensure that any drug selection and dosage set forth in this text are in accordance with current recommendations and practice at the time of publication. However, in view of ongoing research, changes in government regulations, and the constant flow of information relating to drug therapy and drug reactions, the reader is urged to check the package insert for each drug for any change in indications and dosage and for added warnings and precautions. This is particularly important when the recommended agent is a new or infrequently employed drug.

Some drugs and medical devices presented in this publication may have Food and Drug Administration (FDA) clearance for limited use in restricted research settings. It is the responsibility of the health care provider to ascertain the FDA status of each drug or device planned for use in their clinical practice.

Distributed in Canada by Raincoast Books

Copyright © 2008 by R. Keith McCormick, DC
New Harbinger Publications, Inc.
5674 Shattuck Avenue
Oakland, CA 94609
www.newharbinger.com

All Rights Reserved; Printed in the United States of America

Acquired by Jess O'Brien; Cover design by Amy Shoup; Edited by Kayla Sussell

---

Library of Congress Cataloging-in-Publication Data
McCormick, R. Keith.
 The whole-body approach to osteoporosis : how to improve bone strength and reduce your fracture risk / R. Keith McCormick.
   p. cm.
Includes bibliographical references.
ISBN-13: 978-1-57224-595-2 (pbk. : alk. paper)
ISBN-10: 1-57224-595-6 (pbk. : alk. paper)
 1. Osteoporosis--Prevention--Popular works. I. Title.
RC931.O73M396 2009
616.7'16--dc22

                        2009007130

16 15 14   10 9 8 7 6 5 4

To Ty and Colten, my daily reminders to strive for a strong, healthy body.

Contents

Acknowledgments

There are four special people from New Harbinger Publications whom I would like to acknowledge. The idea for this book would not have been born without Wendy Millstine, acquistions editor. I am indebted to Wendy for her unwavering belief in me. Thank you to Kayla Sussell, whose expertise and painstaking copy editing efforts helped bring the book to full fruition. A heartfelt thank-you to Jasmine Star, proofreader extraordinaire, and to Heather Mitchener, editorial director, for contributing so much to this book's readability.

This book would not have been possible without the constant encouragement, endless late nights of dedication, and fine attention to concept and detail of my local editor, Elizabeth Earl Phillips. Thank you, Liz.

Many thanks go to my patients who have inspired my studies of bone biology and osteoporosis and especially to those who have personally encouraged me over the past year during the writing of this book. And thank you to Christine Purcell, my office manager, for putting up with my constant writing and inattention to business matters.

I would like to extend a very special thank-you to Mary Ann Page and John Clayton, who so graciously offered to read this manuscript and suggest organizational and editorial changes.

Thank you to Paul Rezendes for his teachings and deep friendship, and to his wife Paulette Roy for her help and support when I was in the first stages of preparing to undertake this project.

I extend my sincerest appreciation to Christy Maxwell, MS; Eve Bralley, Ph.D.; Jeffery Moss, DDS; Tom O'Bryan, DC; and Ted Czepiel, DC; for their literary research and professional suggestions. Thank you also to Nancy Haver for your wonderful illustrations.

Special thanks go to my good friend, Kara Fitzgerald, ND, for her generosity with time and her invariable willingness to discuss complex scientific issues. Kara's brilliance brought substantial depth to this book.

And, finally, I would like to express profound thanks to my wife, Eva Lohrer, for her patience around the hours and hours of time I needed to complete this book and to my two sons, Ty for his encouragement and Colten for the endless games of floor hockey that kept me sane.

Introduction

Each time I walk into the woods I find myself wandering off the trail. This habit comes from years of mentoring by my friend Paul Rezendes, a tracker and nature photographer in New England, who taught me the finer points of tracking animals through the forest. Of all his teachings, the most important was how to look beyond the forest trails left by humans and see into worlds that few ever see. He taught me to track an animal from just the slightest disturbance to stone or twig or scent and to not only open my eyes to the forest's beauty but to touch its very soul. Paul is able to see the forest through the microvision of a mole's eye, yet in the same instant he can see its intricate matrix like a hawk soaring above the treetops. This is how he taught me to look—so I could see. Now when I enter a forest, I sense it differently. My eyes and ears are somehow more open, more receptive to its whispers of beauty and grace.

The approach I take to tracking down the causes for osteoporosis largely stems from these teachings. In certain ways, evaluating a patient can be similar to entering a new forest. It's easy to stay on the trails and look at what everyone else is looking at, but step off the trail, look, listen, and poke around, and you begin to sense the real forest. Similarly, when evaluating someone for bone loss, it's easy to look for the obvious, but if you begin to search through every nook and cranny of a person's physiology, listening for valuable connections between the person's symptoms and looking for subtleties and trends in his or her laboratory tests, it's possible to find reasons for bone loss that might go undetected in traditional diagnostic evaluations.

In the same way that Paul was my mentor in tracking nature through the forest, I would like to be your mentor and show you a unique way to track bone loss through the forest of your physiology. I will not only show you the established protocol for diagnosis and treatment of osteoporosis, I will also take you off the traditional trails of medical thinking and teach you how to explore your own physiology. You will learn to find the hidden factors for your bone loss and to reduce your risk for fracture.

WHY A WHOLE-BODY APPROACH TO OSTEOPOROSIS?

Osteoporosis is a chronic disorder. It's not a condition you can fix by swallowing a daily or weekly pill, or even by a yearly intravenous infusion of an extremely powerful bone-specific medication. Unfortunately, in our country the same approach used to treat acute conditions is also used with chronic disorders such as osteoporosis. For example, in crisis care management, the doctor visually examines a patient, possibly scrapes for a culture or analyzes the patient's blood, and then prescribes a pill or a shot to reduce the symptoms. The underlying physiological vulnerability is usually never questioned—let alone assessed. The patient feels better, the crisis is satisfactorily averted, and yet the nutrient deficiency or physiological dysfunction that might eventually damage his or her long-term health is not addressed and stays unchanged.

Pharmaceuticals for osteoporosis can be extremely valuable, but they are overprescribed and almost never used as they should be—as an adjunct to a solid therapeutic protocol based on nutrition and lifestyle. To help someone with a chronic condition, that person's whole physiology must be assessed and a plan made to restore their failing biological functions. And it can be done. Optimal skeletal health can be achieved through the use of nutrition and exercise. In such a program, medications are best used to bail out the person from a bad situation.

Osteoporosis is not just the weakening of bones; it is a weakening of the body's entire physiology. To put it more accurately, a weakened physiology leads to bone loss and requires a broader evaluation than just an assessment of bone. When you have a chronic disease, you have to treat your whole body.

BARE BONES OF OSTEOPOROSIS

Your bones not only provide you with structural support, they also serve as storage vessels for the key minerals calcium and phosphorous. When you break apart a chicken bone, you see the central cavity is filled with fatty marrow. This is where the white blood cells of the immune system and the oxygen-carrying red blood cells are formed. Keeping your skeleton healthy is important both to prevent fractures and to maintain your bone marrow's vigorous cell production.

The statistics for poor bone health are daunting. Over 10 million Americans have been diagnosed with osteoporosis. As the word "osteoporosis" suggests, this metabolic disease is characterized by porous, weakened bone with a low mass and a deterioration of its microarchitecture. This reduction in both quantity and quality is caused by nutrient deficiency or a systemic dysfunction that lead to fragility and a greater risk for fracture. Amazingly, 30 to 50 percent of women and 13 to 30 percent of men will sustain an osteoporosis-related fracture in their lifetime (Chrischilles et al. 1991).

Most of these fractures occur in the spine (vertebrae), forearm (radius), or hip (femur). Spinal fractures are extremely common and can lead to chronic pain and a disfiguring forward-stooped posture that reduces the individual's heart and lung capacity. Hip fractures often lead to long-term disability and, due to complications, even death. Each year 1.5 million people in the United States sustain an osteoporosis-related fracture (Riggs and Melton 1995). But it does not have to be this way.

It is clear that, for some, osteoporosis treatment should have begun with prevention. Years of suboptimal nutrition and a failure to reach peak bone mass during childhood and early adulthood (the time when bone is genetically programmed to reach its maximum mineral content and strength) will increase a person's risk for fracture later in life. But not all osteoporosis is the result of poor nutrition, and prevention is not always possible. Osteoporosis can sneak up on anyone, seemingly coming from out of nowhere.

If you are reading this book, in all probability you've been diagnosed with either osteopenia or osteoporosis and are searching for ways to help reduce your fracture risk. You have come to the right source, and by taking a whole body approach to osteoporosis, you will find very concrete ways to help yourself.

WHICH APPROACH WILL YOU CHOOSE?

Suffering a fracture from minimal trauma or discovering that your bone density is deficient are the usual gateways to the world of osteoporosis. Whichever your introduction, the therapeutic focus of most physicians is often directed at improving one thing only—your bone density. Most physicians prescribe pharmaceuticals along with an extra helping of calcium and vitamin D as quick and easy therapy for osteoporosis. The need to address the disease process that underlies your bone loss is frequently ignored. This approach lacks the sophistication required to match the complexity of this disease process. If you plan to live with your bones for years to come, they need more than just to be made harder; they need to become healthier.

If you prefer a more natural healing approach, you can work to remedy your bone loss by way of dietary modifications, weight-bearing exercises, and bone-healthy recipes. But how will you know which supplements to take? There are scores of nutrients necessary for bone health, and claims of magic bullets for osteoporosis abound in health magazines and on the Internet. Without being able to see into the forest of your physiology, how can you know what your bones need? And how can you know if what you're taking is working?

You are facing difficult decisions about what course of treatment to follow. Unfortunately, the huge amount of available information can be confusing and it's easy to become overwhelmed. When you're already burdened with concern or even fear of the disease, it sometimes may be difficult to think straight. Every forest is difficult to navigate, especially if you lack the skills to make your way through. I'm sure you agree with me that neither confusion nor fear is a good reason for making a possibly life-altering decision.

Luckily, there is another approach to osteoporosis—one through which you can view your physiological landscape and systematically determine what is needed to improve the health of your bones. It is a method in which information from two sources is gathered to determine therapeutic targets to guide treatment. The first source is your own assessment of your physical signs and symptoms. Your body may show signs of physiological dysfunction, or you may experience symptoms for which neither you nor your doctor can find a cause. I often have new patients tell me of symptoms that have troubled them for years about which their primary care doctors had been unconcerned. Such symptoms may have great utility. They may offer clues to understand the cause of your bone loss and, by their remedy, may offer a way to gain better health.

The second source of information is the results of standard laboratory tests, called *biomarkers*, which can be ordered by your doctor. Objective measures of organ dysfunction and metabolic error can serve as monitors to help you modify your lifestyle, diet, and supplemental nutrition in order to help your whole physiology. And that which improves physiology improves bone. Using targeted laboratory biomarkers will enable you to look beyond the traditional boundaries of medical diagnostic and therapeutic "trails" toward an individualized approach for defining and positively altering your specific biochemical identity.

It's more than likely that your bone loss is just one symptom of a greater story of ill health—one that must be approached through a sophisticated, evidence-based platform. This book offers a manageable step-by-step process that will first take you off trail into the physiology of your bone loss and then hand you a map to bring you home in better health. This is how I would approach osteoporosis if I had it—which, in fact, I do.

MY PERSONAL EXPERIENCE WITH OSTEOPOROSIS

When I was forty five years old, I became lame with hip pain while running a track workout. After an MRI, hip X-rays, a bone scan, and finally a bone-mineral density evaluation, I was diagnosed with many small fractures in my hip and severe osteoporosis. At that point, I didn't understand the serious significance of a T score of -4.3. (A *T score* is the number calculated from a bone density examination used to determine the risk of fracture.) But I should have caught on when the technician blurted, "Wow, you have worse bone density than a hundred-year-old woman!"

My first reaction was embarrassment. How could I have this? I'd eaten well all my life; or at least I thought I had. I'd always drunk a lot of milk. I'd never smoked, drunk alcohol, or used any type of drug or medication. I'd never done anything "wrong." I'd always done everything "right" to be healthy. It just didn't make any sense. Osteoporosis—a disease associated with frailty—was the antithesis of who I thought I was. From early on, the foundation of my life centered on developing the strongest, fastest, healthiest body I could. I had always wanted to be an Olympian, and it seemed that from day one my attitude had been one of wanting to improve—to be the best, strongest, toughest competitor out there. My body was the vessel by which to achieve this, and I had fueled it with those goals in mind.

I didn't tell anyone of my condition. I was too embarrassed—ashamed of what I had become—a broken-down old man in what I had thought was the prime of my life.

Initially, I struggled, not knowing how I was going to get out of this crumbling skeletal mess. Before I was diagnosed, I felt that I was almost unstoppable and certainly unbreakable. Osteoporosis did *not* fit with my unbreakable self-image. Now I was afraid I would fracture my spine if I opened the garage door or bent down to pick up something, and certainly shatter if I fell off my bike. Always one to help out at my sons' school, moving benches, lifting boxes, building sheds, I began to hide or made excuses. I was supposed to be strong, an Ironman (triathlete), an ex-Olympian no less. And now, just like that, I couldn't move a table. Everyone would surely think I was a wimp!

The voice of the orthopedist, "You should go on disability" and "Now promise me that you'll walk with a cane," made me want to throw up. When I stood before a mirror, no matter how long I searched for that person I used to be, all I saw was emptiness. My self-confidence, as well as my inner structural core, had withered away.

If you were recently diagnosed with osteoporosis, you may be going through an adjustment period similar to mine. This is natural and very common among those who have just learned that they are at high risk for breaking their hip or spine. It's scary, and the reality is that no one can definitively predict what your real risk for fracturing is. This makes it hard to know what your limits are, and it's easy to become overly fearful of movements. Doing the things you once did without thinking now makes you anxious and concerned. This is normal.

The first endocrinologist I saw read down a list of about twenty diseases that can cause severe bone loss, asking me questions after each item. When he got to the bottom of the list, he diagnosed me with primary osteoporosis and handed me two prescriptions. One was for a thiazide diuretic, to help reduce the calcium loss in my urine, and the other for alendronate (Fosamax), a bisphosphonate to harden my bones. I told him that I wasn't there for prescriptions—I was there to find out *why* I had osteoporosis—and to fix it.

After calls and e-mails to three more endocrinologists, one of whom wrote back asking for the date of my last menstrual period, I finally made an appointment with one who specialized in the treatment of osteoporosis. The day of my appointment came and, as I opened the door to his waiting room, I stepped into a world that made me shudder. Trying to look invisible, I walked slowly to a chair and sat down. There were three other patients: all older women, all in wheelchairs, each with a dowager's hump indicating spinal degeneration from a series of compression fractures. All three women looked downward. They did not speak. They did not make eye contact with me or each other. Each was withdrawn as though she were collapsing inward. And then it dawned on me. These women were now my peers.

When I left that office, I never looked back. I was on a mission—a mission not only to find out everything I could about my osteoporosis and fix it, but also to gain back my lost self-confidence. It is a loss that you too may be feeling, especially if your osteoporosis is severe and you've already broken some bones.

WHY I WROTE THIS BOOK

When I was first diagnosed, I wished I had a manual to study. With no instructions to guide me, my mission proved difficult and I suffered more than a few setbacks. Over the five years immediately following my diagnosis, I experienced twelve *fragility fractures* (broken bones that result from minimal trauma)—but I also learned a lot about osteoporosis. Other than being told by the endocrinologists to take calcium supplements and drink milk, I was given no nutritional recommendations by my doctors. They were excellent and painstaking in their diagnostic process, ensuring that no other disease was involved in my body's secret weakening of its bones. They were caring, thorough, and positive.

But their training was completely within the realm of pharmaceuticals. The doctors had little or no experience with using nutrition as therapy. And they did not understand that it was actually possible to use nutrition to influence patients' physiology so profoundly that not only could their bones become less fragile but their blood and urine laboratory biomarkers would be altered as proof of their improvement. But at that time, neither did I.

It was only after painstaking research and a thorough process of trial and error that I discovered the value of using laboratory biomarkers to design and monitor the nutritional treatment for my osteoporosis. Later, I began using these same methods to help my patients with their bone loss. This proved to be a great improvement over using nutrition in a hit-or-miss approach to skeletal health. In patients with severe osteoporosis, it was the merger of nutrition with pharmaceuticals that provided a much greater reduction in fracture risk than that which was attainable through drug therapy alone. In addition, the patient's overall health was greatly improved—a secondary benefit that never would have been attained otherwise.

My goal in writing this book is twofold. I want to provide you with a user-friendly manual bursting with information to empower you and enhance your life. I also want to offer you hope and understanding. I've been there. I have been exactly where you are right now, facing the unknown, confronting a disease process that can destroy your freedom to move for fear of breaking your bones. So, I encourage you—don't give up. There are many positive actions you can take to effectively build your bone strength and reduce your fracture risk. There is not only hope; there are answers.

This book is the manual I had wished for.

The Organization of This Book

The book is organized to be read from front to back. Each chapter will provide you with a higher level of understanding and will help you to see the big picture of whole-body wellness necessary for skeletal health. Throughout the chapters you'll find interactive exercises that require your thoughtful attention. Some of these exercises ask you to do some writing. For that reason, purchasing a full-size notebook specifically to work with these written exercises is highly recommended. That way you will have plenty of room to write down your answers, which also can serve as a valuable record of your treatment plans over time.

COMMITMENT

Making the lifestyle changes required to improve your skeletal health is difficult, but with patience, it can be done. It's a step-by-step process that demands time, financial commitment, and considerable effort. However, in the end, the recovery of your health will be worth it. By adventuring off the well-traveled diagnostic and therapeutic trails, you will discover valuable approaches to improve your bone health and you will also gain a broader vision of the many ways you have to improve your overall health and well-being—indeed, your life.

So, from this moment on, take responsibility for your health. Be positive and try not to let setbacks get you down. Focus on what you need to do to cast aside the shackles of the physical limitations some-times imposed by this disease. Now is the time to commit to yourself and make your skeleton your life's internal stronghold. You are worth it.

CHAPTER ONE

Bone Biology and the Imbalance That Leads to Osteoporosis

Admit it! Go ahead, 'fess up. If you have low bone density and especially if you are as desperate as I was to climb out of that pit of osteoporosis, on occasion you've downed way too much calcium. If it was in tablet form, you got terrible abdominal bloating and so much gas that nobody wanted to stay in the same room with you. If it was in capsule form, you may have experienced the dreaded osteoporosis "dragon burp." That's when your desperation led, not to a belching puff of foul odor and scorching flames, but to the embarrassingly creepy, spontaneous discharge of pulverized white calcium.

We all know calcium is important for bone health, but it's not as simple as ingesting more of it and hoping for a positive effect on your skeleton. If you understand how your bones are put together and why they fall apart, you'll be better equipped to make sensible decisions about your skeletal health and avoid unseemly dragon burps.

THE SKELETON: THE CORE OF YOUR EXISTENCE

At the risk of overstating its importance, I might speak of your skeleton not as just your structural support but as the core of your existence. Had you been born boneless, you would be but a glob of flesh and guts. Literally, you could not survive without your bones. They act both as structural supports that give your body form and as metabolic vessels—crucibles, if you will—where vital minerals are held in reserve and red blood cells and immune system cells are made within their marrow, just like that inside of chicken bones.

The dual function that bone serves, providing your body with a structural foundation while simultaneously being a repository of the minerals necessary for life, is a conflict in job description that, unfortunately, often leads to bone loss. When you are healthy and can adequately attain and absorb nutrients, your skeleton's dual function is preserved and works well. But when your body is struggling and nutrients are scarce, minerals essential for energy production and the growth of tissues (life's key metabolic activities) are tapped from your bones at the expense of maintaining their strength. This is what you are trying to avoid.

The Composite Structure of Bone

Bone is a connective tissue, similar in a way to other tissues of the body such as skin or your ligaments and tendons. But your bones have an added component: they are impregnated with minerals to make them stiff. The fibrous foundation of bone, called the *matrix,* meaning mother or womb, is predominately made of a specialized collagen protein. This incredibly tough fiber is wound like a braid to make it even stronger and then is laced with other proteins, enzymes, and cell-signaling molecules called *cytokines*, all of which are necessary to keep bone alive and healthy. It's through mineralization of the matrix that bone takes on its properties as a stiff structure that supports the transmission of muscular power and as the organ that stores mineral reserves. These reserves consist mainly of calcium and phosphate crystals, which combine to form *hydroxyapatite*. This mineral complex bonds tightly to the collagen fibers like a glue and makes them rigid and strong.

Bone is a composite structure organized in two layers (see figure 1-1). *Compact* bone forms the hard outer *cortex*, or exterior, of the bone. For bone to be strong, this cortex is very dense and built like the tubular walls of a bicycle frame. These walls are of sufficient thickness and density to resist bending and twisting forces but not so thick as to weigh you down and prevent you from getting up a hill. In the *medullary cavity* of bone (the central part), where the marrow is located, there is a more fragile and spongy, or *cancellous*, bone that developed the best of lightness and strength that natural selection could provide. The *trabeculae* are a lattice of three-dimensional structural beams, like a honeycomb, that gives cancellous bone its ability to be featherweight yet tough. Trabeculae should be plentiful, robust, and fully intact to help maintain the strength and form of the bone's outer cortical sheath. Our survival as a species depends upon this compact-cancellous composite of bone.

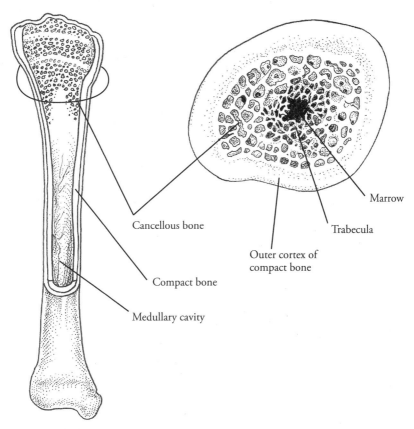

FIGURE 1-1: The structure of bone.

BONE REMODELING: REPAIR AND RENEWAL

In order to maintain a strong, healthy skeleton throughout your life, both compact and cancellous bone undergo periods of repair through a complicated renewal process called *remodeling*. This process ensures a continual replacement of old bone, weakened by microfractures caused by daily activity, with new bone. This highly orchestrated remodeling process involves three different types of bone cells and their precursors (see figure 1-2).

Osteoclasts are the bone-resorbing cells. When osteoclasts resorb bone, they do not actually absorb it again as this word seems to imply, but simply break it down during the remodeling process. The osteoclasts break down old, worn, and weakened bone by secreting acidic chemicals and then ingesting the debris. These bone cells are fairly large, as cells go, and highly mobile. Complex chemical signaling from an area in need of remodeling attracts smaller cells from the bloodstream, which are the precursors to these larger osteoclast cells.

Precursor cells are intermediate cells that have started the differentiation process from stem cells and have committed their development to a certain specialized cell type, but have not yet reached full maturity. In other words, precursor cells are halfway between a stem cell and a specialized cell. The precursors or osteoclasts congregate into areas of accumulated microfractures, where they fuse together to form mature osteoclasts with many nuclei that are capable of resorbing bone.

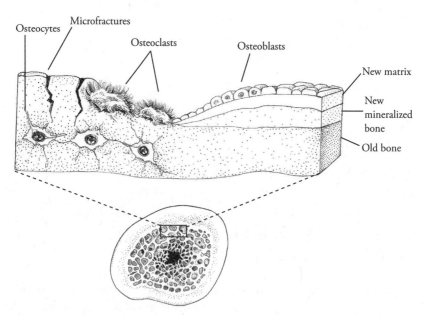

FIGURE 1-2: A magnified view of sectioned trabeculae in cancellous bone undergoing remodeling.

Osteoblasts are the bone-forming cells. Immature osteoblasts, or pre-osteoblasts, also migrate to areas of needed repair, but because they are formed within the bone itself, they don't have far to travel to those areas. The osteoblasts mature once they reach the tunneled-out area of bone recently resorbed by the osteoclasts, and there they deposit new collagen matrix that will eventually become strong mineralized bone. As long as the remodeling process is needed, precursors to osteoblasts are constantly being summoned to the area. As these pre-osteoblasts approach, they brush against cells that are the precursors of osteoclasts (the pre-osteoclasts) and release a molecule called *RANKL* (see figure 1-3). This signaling molecule activates the pre-osteoclasts, causing them to mature and resorb more bone as needed. The actions between the two cell types (osteoclasts and osteoblasts) are closely linked and are referred to as a *coupled process* that is kept in balance by a third cell, the osteocyte.

Osteocytes, the supervisors or foremen, orchestrate the entire complicated remodeling process. Osteocytes are embedded within the bone matrix and, through extended armlike appendages called *canaliculi*, are able to sense microcracks in bone. Once there is enough microdamage requiring repair, the osteocytes initiate localized areas of remodeling through a series of signals and messages carried by the cytokines to activate hormonal release.

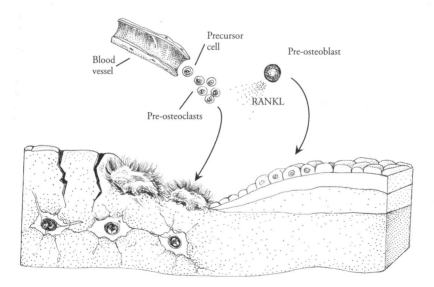

FIGURE 1-3: RANKL being released by pre-osteoblasts to couple remodeling activity with that of the pre-osteoclasts and mature osteoclasts.

At any one moment 2 to 5 percent of your skeleton is being remodeled. Right now, there are millions of these tiny areas of bone undergoing active repair in your body. These localized demolition-construction sites of coupled remodeling are referred to as *basic multicellular units*. The osteoclastic resorption phase of remodeling lasts for three to five weeks, and the osteoblastic bone formation and subsequent mineralization phase takes another three to five months to complete.

WHAT LEADS TO BONE LOSS?

During the remodeling process it is important to have a balance between the amount of bone being resorbed by the osteoclasts and that which is formed by the osteoblasts. A negative balance, where resorption exceeds formation in what is called an *uncoupled remodeling process*, results in a net bone loss. If this uncoupled process becomes chronic, it will lead to osteoporosis. This imbalance in an uncoupled remodeling process can be from increased resorption, decreased formation, or a combination of the two. The underlying abnormalities that contribute to this disequilibrium and the therapeutic measures by which they are corrected are what you will be learning about throughout this book.

When we compare normal to osteoporotic bone (figure 1-4), it is easy to see why the osteoporotic bone is more fragile. Its cortex (the outer sheath of bone) is attenuated and the trabeculae have become rodlike, spindly, and scarce. Some of the trabeculae are completely disconnected; they look like microscopic stalactites and stalagmites and offer absolutely no structural support to the bone. Even when density is added through osteoporosis medications, the trabecular stubs never reunite and they remain structurally ineffective. This is where the hope of reduced fracture risk through improved density with bisphosphonates (the medications most commonly prescribed for the treatment of osteoporosis) is sometimes overly optimistic. Why? Because although additional bone is being made, that new bone is not structurally sound.

Bone mineral density begins to decline even before mid-adulthood. In women, this means that bone loss may begin before estrogen levels start to recede at menopause. Nothing is wrong with this if the loss is slight and gradual, especially if the person reached peak bone mass as a young adult. But many of us encounter a complication during our lives that seems only to worsen as we age, and that is chronic low-level inflammation.

Normal bone   Osteoporotic bone

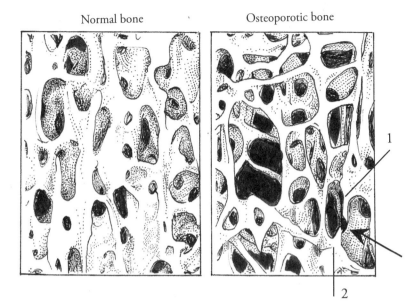

FIGURE 1-4: Normal bone compared to osteoporotic bone. Notice the disconnected trabecula (arrow) with its stalactite (1) and stalagmite (2) appearance in the lower right corner of the osteoporotic bone.

Chronic Low-Level Inflammation

We are all familiar with acute inflammation. We cut ourselves, we fall and our skin gets scraped, or we catch a cold and get a fever. In all these situations the symptoms are the same: redness, heat, pain, and swelling. These are the classic signs of inflammation. They are the signs that the body's immune system is responding to the stress of injury. Whether the assault is traumatic or microbial in origin, the response is very much the same. *Acute inflammation* is the body's way of initiating its defense against invading organisms, walling them off from doing damage to other body parts, and finally promoting healing. The immune system's inflammatory response is vital to survival.

But if this response continues for months or years, instead of being reparative, the immune system becomes unbalanced and destructive to the body. Conditions such as long-term infection, exposure to toxins, food allergies, vitamin D deficiency, abnormal overgrowth of bacteria within the gut, or even constant emotional stress can create undue pressure on the immune system. As you will read in greater depth in chapter 4, this distress leads to chronic low-level inflammation, a major component of many chronic diseases, including osteoporosis.

If you had asked me before my diagnosis if I thought I was healthy, I would certainly have replied, yes. But when I started to research osteoporosis and began finding huge amounts of information spelling out the relationship between bone loss and its connection to inflammation and the immune system, I began to see constitutional signs that I'd never paid attention to before. Signs and symptoms I had ignored for years suggested that my physiology had indeed hinted at nutrient deficiency, immune system distress, and inflammation—signs that a riptide of destructive forces was probably destroying me from the inside out.

Chronic vs. Acute Inflammation

Chronic inflammation is different from the inflammation of an acute injury. Its intensity level is lower and the body doesn't display the same classic signs of agony: redness, heat, pain, and swelling. Chronic inflammation may not shout out and wave a red flag at you. You may have to learn to recognize its presence. Skin sensitivity, irritability, anger, fatigue, depression, general stiffness, nagging joint pain—these were some of my warnings. Start listening to your own. Don't just pass them off as an unfortunate part of aging. Chronic low-level inflammation is important to recognize—it is key to understanding bone loss—and there's a lot you can do to diminish its destructive forces.

The Destructive Forces of Catabolism

All of us have some inflammation. It helps us to heal from injuries and defends us from pathogens in our environment. But an overabundance of inflammation is a curse, not a blessing. It's a backdrop for ill health and eventually leads to a body that destroys itself—that is, a body with a catabolic physiology. *Catabolism* is the destructive breakdown of complex molecules in the body—a classic description of someone with osteoporosis.

I should have seen it earlier. Besides the signs of inflammation, my muscles seemed more flaccid than when I was younger. Instead of winning races, I was struggling to finish them. My V-shaped muscular physique had deteriorated to that of a withered scarecrow on a bleak November day. Muscle wasting and the reduced ability to build or repair tissue is a sign of a catabolic physiology. Silently beneath the muscles, the bone too wastes away. Simply taking calcium and vitamin D and engaging in weight-bearing exercise, although helpful, will not match the overpowering destructive nature of chronic inflammation.

The opposite of catabolic is *anabolic*, which refers to the constructive synthesis and repair of the body. Throughout this book we will focus on making your body more anabolic: encouraging a healthy digestive system able to absorb vitamins, minerals, and proteins; promoting a body free of inflammatory stressors; and neutralizing the body's pH (its amount of acidity or alkalinity) for proper enzymatic function and mineral balance. When these are all present, we foster an anabolic physiology capable of healing. Without them, chronic disease and the destructive processes of a catabolic physiology persist.

WHAT IS THE LEVEL OF YOUR HEALTH?

To be healthy, your skeleton requires the same good things as the rest of your body, but with the addition of a lot more calcium. So if you aren't healthy, there's a fairly good chance that your bones aren't healthy either. As you age, it's easy to settle into your body even if it's not feeling that great. Health recedes slowly and frailty has a way of sneaking up on you without notice. It's like the wear on the soles of your running shoes. You seem to be running fine until one day you pull up lame because your shoes have worn out, as if the soles had somehow broken down overnight while you were sleeping.

But take a moment, look back, and see if there aren't signs or symptoms of erosion. *Signs* are the objective evidence of disease—things that both you and your doctor can detect, such as abdominal distention or bloating. *Symptoms*, on the other hand, can be more elusive, and your doctor might not be able to perceive them even though subjectively you are experiencing them. For example, abdominal pain or feelings of fatigue after eating a particular food are important symptoms that should be evaluated. In the following exercise, you'll take a look at a list of common signs and symptoms. If you regularly experience any of these, they may be signals of ill health—signals indicating that your running shoes could use some maintenance.

The first list calls out symptoms related to nutrient deficiencies. The second list calls out the gastrointestinal and urinary indicators of poor health that may be connected to bone loss. And the third list is a short sampling of what could be a very long list of generalized symptoms indicative of a suboptimal physiology, toxicity, or a state of chronic inflammation.

EXERCISE 1.1: Sign and Symptom Overview

Complete this exercise by highlighting or circling any signs or symptoms you are experiencing.

SIGNS AND SYMPTOMS OF NUTRIENT DEFICIENCIES

Fingernails: Brittle; flattened with raised ridges or depressions; white streaks or spots; chronic soft tissue infection around nail; *psoriatic* (pitted).

Hair: Dry, brittle; thin, lifeless, low luster; easily plucked.

Skin: Bumpy on back of arms; dry, scaly, flaking; seborrhea (scaly, itchy, red skin) in nasal folds alongside nose to corners of mouth; easy bruising (small red or purple spots); psoriasis, eczema, seborrhea, dandruff; dermatitis (inflammation such as with eczema); hypersensitive.

Lips: Cracks at edges of the mouth.

Tongue: Decreased taste or smell; yellow coated; white coated; *glossitis* (swollen, inflamed).

Teeth: Cavities and premature tooth loss; periodontal disease (bleeding, swollen gums).

Muscle: Spasms; weakness.

GASTROINTESTINAL AND URINARY SYMPTOMS

Abdominal: Bloating, prolonged fullness after eating; sensitivity to many foods.

Upper GI tract: Belching.

Lower GI: Constipation; copious gas; pale, foul-smelling stool; pale stool floats in the bowl; sensitive right lower abdomen; diarrhea.

Urinary tract: Frequent urination.

SIGNS AND SYMPTOMS OF POOR SYSTEMIC HEALTH AND TOXICITY

Dark circles under eyes; sensitivity along outside of thigh; chronic morning stiffness; frequent headaches; weight loss; depression, fatigue, anger.

Scoring: Count those problems that you have on a regular basis. It's not good to have any, but if you've checked off three, four, or more, then your body may have more forces at work tearing down its tissues than building them up. If this is the case, you have some work to do. The longer the symptoms have been there and the greater their number, the more likely it is that they indicate serious physiological impairment.

The next list is a short one but it contains three classic signs of a catabolic physiology. You'll note that bone loss is first on the list. Again, mark all that pertain to you.

SIGNS AND SYMPTOMS OF A CATABOLIC (WASTING) PHYSIOLOGY

Osteopenia or osteoporosis (bone loss); sarcopenia (muscle wasting); inability to maintain body weight.

THERAPEUTIC TARGETS

Physical signs and symptoms and abnormal laboratory biomarkers (test results) can be focused on, like targets, to help improve your bone health. Just as you would target the bull's-eye to improve your skills as a competitive marksman, you can target signs, symptoms, and lab tests to improve your therapeutic aim. For example, if you highlighted or circled "abdominal bloating" and "copious gas," these can be used as targets for therapy. These symptoms indicate digestive dysfunction, which may prevent you from absorbing the nutrients necessary for bone health. By establishing the cause of these symptoms, such as a food sensitivity or an insufficient production of hydrochloric acid (HCl) in your stomach, and then taking steps to remedy them, you will affect mechanisms that may be linked to your bone loss. I will explain throughout the book the importance of these various markers.

CHAPTER TWO

Evaluating Bone Loss

If you were a novice hiker embarking on a wilderness trek through uncharted and treacherous terrain, I would hope that you had an experienced knowledgeable companion by your side. Preferably, your guide would be communicative and would include you in all decision making. This expert guide would be attentive to your emotional and physical well-being and would always strive to keep you safe. Similar qualifications should apply to choosing a health care provider. He or she must be knowledgeable, willing to discuss therapeutic options, and capable of helping you navigate the maze of decisions necessary to improve your bone health.

CHOOSING YOUR HEALTH CARE PROVIDER

Many physicians are not expert in the complexities of osteoporosis. They may not fully understand the serious physical and emotional consequences attached to the diagnosis, and they may be unaware of the correlation between osteoporosis and other inflammatory-based chronic conditions, such as cardiovascular disease and Alzheimer's. Physicians often see osteoporosis primarily as a loss of bone density that can be restored only by the use of medications, and they underestimate the necessity for intensive ongoing therapy requiring, as its foundation, nutrition and lifestyle management.

Despite mounting scientific evidence that nutritional therapy is effective in reducing fractures, traditional physicians have been slow to embrace it as a serious first option. Even the basic nutritional recommendations for maintaining bone health, 1,200 mg per day of calcium and

800 IU per day of vitamin D, are rarely mentioned during most medical examinations. This paucity of nutritional awareness was highlighted in a recent study (Kramm and Hansen 2006) demonstrating that even though vitamin D insufficiency is common among doctors themselves, they still do not check the vitamin D levels of their patients.

With these facts in mind, you must choose your health care provider for osteoporosis carefully. That person may be your primary care physician or another provider with more expertise in osteoporosis. In either case, you will be working with this person on your "wilderness trek" for years to come. Preferably your guide will be knowledgeable about osteoporosis and, more importantly, will have training and experience in nutrition. There are many chiropractic physicians, naturopaths, medical doctors, osteopaths, and clinical nutritionists whose practices emphasize the general restoration of health and function in addition to addressing distinct disorders. Some practitioners have specialized training in functional or integrative medicine that emphasizes a holistic approach to chronic disease. Here are the Web addresses of two organizations that may be helpful in locating a provider with this expertise: the Institute for Functional Medicine at Gig Harbor in Washington can be reached at www.functionalmedicine.org, and the American Academy of Naturopathic Physicians in Washington, DC, can be accessed at www.naturopathic.org.

It is most important that your clinician take the time required to provide you with good quality care. This can't happen in a fifteen-minute appointment or without some basic laboratory testing. If you aren't satisfied with your current clinician, ask friends, go online, do some research, and look for a health care provider who will be able to meet your needs. Don't be afraid to call a doctor's office to talk to him or her on the phone for a while before making an appointment. All good doctors should be willing to spend a few minutes to explain their approach to osteoporosis.

MEASURING BONE MINERAL DENSITY

If you haven't already had a bone density examination, this is one of the first tests your doctor will order. Skeletal health is quantified by means of a simple, painless procedure called a *dual-energy X-ray absorptiometry (DXA) examination*. Its objective is to determine the level of your bone mineral density (BMD).

Dual-Energy X-ray Absorptiometry

Bone densitometry is the gold standard for defining bone loss and determining fracture risk. If your density is low, you are at greater risk for breaking a bone. Every bone is vulnerable, but those most commonly fractured are the spinal vertebrae, ribs, forearms, and hip bones. When density is exceptionally low, it doesn't take much trauma to break something. If you're osteoporotic, it's not uncommon to fracture a rib just by sneezing or a vertebra by opening a garage door or leaning down to pick up a dirty sock. Knowing the level of your bone density is a valuable part of understanding the extent to which you are vulnerable to fracture.

If you've had a bone density scan, you probably wondered what the machine was doing as it "hummed" back and forth across your body. This is what was happening: From inside the table underneath you, a very small amount of radiation (electromagnetic waves) was being emitted. As the X-ray beam passed through your body, it was partially blocked, attenuated, or weakened, by the minerals inside your skeleton. The scanner roving above your body was measuring the electromagnetic energy that was not being blocked. Like a matrix printer that spells out the pixels of a document, the DXA spells out the mineral substance of your bones. The radiation that passes through is affected by your body's mineral content. The more minerals present in your bones, the more dense and capable they are at blocking this radiation—and at resisting fracture. The degree of attenuation is calculated and measured in units of grams for a specified area of bone. For the purpose of fracture-risk comparison, this information is converted into T and Z scores.

T AND Z SCALES AND SCORES

There are two separate scoring systems on a DXA report: the T and Z scores. Both scales are used to indicate how your bone density compares to that of others. *T scores* are a value of measurement that compares your BMD to that of a healthy young woman. The *Z scale* compares your bone density to that of people your same age and sex. In 1994, a World Health Organization (WHO) study group defined *osteoporosis* as a deterioration in the quality of bone and quantified the definition as requiring a bone density T score of -2.5 standard deviations below that of the bone density of a healthy, young, white female.

A *standard deviation* is the measurement of variation of bone density around an average value found in healthy people. So the difference between the amount of bone mass found in your skeleton and that found in the skeleton of a person with a healthy amount of bone mass can be designated as *x* standard deviations away, plus or minus, from this average value found in healthy adults. For simplicity's sake, I will use only the T scale throughout this book.

THE WORLD HEALTH ORGANIZATION CLASSIFICATION OF T SCORES

These are the WHO's classifications for T scores: *normal* is a BMD greater than or equal to -1.0; *low bone mass (osteopenia)* is between -2.5 and -1.0; *osteoporosis* is a BMD of -2.5 or less; and *severe (established) osteoporosis* is classified as having a BMD of -2.5 or less with a history of fragility fractures.

Although the WHO study group designated a T score of -2.5 as defining osteoporosis, keep in mind that the risk of fracture is a continuum. A score of -2.5 is simply a way to classify the disease and not a set number that means you will fracture. For example, a T score of -2.4, which is considered *osteopenia*, holds about the same fracture risk as a score of -2.6, which is considered *osteoporosis*. Having low bone density, whether it is -2.4 or -2.6, increases your risk for fracture, but it does not necessarily mean that you are going to fracture. Standard practice estimates that for every standard deviation reduction in T score, your fracture risk approximately doubles.

■ *Ms. Hart*

To understand BMD better, let's look at the test results for Ms. Hart. She is a fifty-year-old secretary who came into my office for a consultation about her low bone density. Her first DXA scan, done five years earlier when she was forty-five, showed she was osteopenic with a T scores of -2.3 at her spine and -1.4 at her hips. If Ms. Hart's T score had been between 1.0 and -1.0, this would be considered normal and indicate an average risk for fracture. But with her low T scores, Ms. Hart had twice the chance of fracturing as someone with normal density.

Now, after five years, a follow-up DXA examination indicated that her spine BMD had fallen to -2.8 and her hips to -1.6. Because of her new scores, Ms. Hart was now considered osteoporotic; her fracture risk was rated approximately three to four times higher than someone with a normal density measurement. If Ms. Hart's bone density continued to fall a full standard deviation to -3.8, her risk would double again to eight times that of a healthy individual.

WHAT DOES A SMALL CHANGE IN DENSITY MEAN?

If you've had more than one DXA examination, you probably noted a change in your T score. Note that it's important to compare only scores obtained from the same machine at the same facility. Different machines have different calibrations and different radiologists interpret data slightly differently. Bone density, especially in postmenopausal women, can even change slightly with the seasons of the year (Need et al. 2007). Depending on your amount of exposure to the sun, your vitamin D levels fluctuate and thus affect your bone density. So when you have repeat exams, it's important to go to the same facility at roughly the same time of the year. Keep all of the variables the same and you will ensure greater reliability and significance of your scores in future examinations.

A follow-up DXA scan must change by at least 3 percent to indicate a true change in BMD. For example, a decrease in T score from -2.8 to -2.9 is too small to be meaningful. A drop to -3.1 or lower would be needed to detect a true loss of density. Of course, this same rule applies when you see improvements in your score. Try not to be overly optimistic if your bone density improves by only a tenth of a standard deviation. On the other hand, an increase from -2.8 to -2.6 should at least be encouraging.

IS THE DXA SCAN SAFE?

A DXA scan is extremely safe. The radiation emitted is minimal. The dose to your body when having a *central scan*, or spine and hip DXA measurement, is between 1 and 5 sieverts of x-radiation. (The *sievert* is a measurement that tries to reflect the biological effects of radiation as opposed to the physical aspects.) Compare this to a mammogram, which is approximately 450 sieverts, or a lateral lumbar spine X-ray, at 700 sieverts. Actually, just being alive on this earth for one day exposes you to between 5 and 8 sieverts of x-radiation (Genant et al. 1996).

VERTEBRAL FRACTURE ASSESSMENT

If you've experienced either a loss in height or your upper back has curved forward into a hunched position, then it's important not only to have a DXA scan, but also to be assessed for spinal compression fractures. These fractures can be silent, often causing no discomfort at all, but identifying them is important. A confirmed osteoporosis-related spinal compression fracture requires pharmaceutical intervention (in addition to nutritional therapy) to help prevent further fracture—no matter what your T score is.

Depending on the circumstances, your doctor may order either a *vertebral fracture assessment* (VFA) or a regular X-ray evaluation of your spine. A VFA is a separate test performed by a DXA machine and is often obtained along with your BMD examination. A VFA allows your doctor to look for compression fractures in your spine without subjecting you to spinal X-rays, which have two hundred times the radiation and cost four times as much.

OTHER WAYS TO ASSESS BONE MINERAL DENSITY

Other technologies are available for evaluating bone loss. For example, a *peripheral DXA,* as opposed to a central DXA exam, and an ultrasound evaluation may be used to screen the forearm, the heel, or a finger. Unfortunately, the BMD in your extremities may not mirror that in your spine or hips. Bone mineral density varies throughout your skeleton, and the amount in your heel may be different than that in your spine. Because a spine or hip fracture has the potential to cause the greatest negative impact on your life, knowing the density of these crucial structures makes the most practical sense. If you haven't already been evaluated by central DXA, ask your doctor.

UNDERSTANDING YOUR DIAGNOSIS

After quantifying your bone density, the next step is to evaluate your risk factors and make a diagnosis. Bone loss that cannot be attributed to another disease process is diagnosed as *primary osteoporosis* and then identified as *type I* for age-related bone loss, *type II* when associated with menopause, or *idiopathic* when seen in younger individuals.

Risk Factors for Primary Osteoporosis

The following list calls out the factors correlated to an increased risk for osteoporosis. As you can see, several factors are completely out of your control. You can't change your age or family history, for example. As you age, you will lose bone density, and there is definitely a genetic link to osteoporosis. But other factors are under your control and can be eliminated through changes in your lifestyle.

These are the risk factors: chronic depression; eating disorders (anorexia nervosa, bulimia); family history of a first-degree relative with osteoporosis; in men, delayed puberty, diminished libido, erectile dysfunction, low testosterone; in women, late menarche, loss of or irregular menstrual periods, or early menopause (estrogen deficiency); low body weight (less than 127 pounds); maternal history of hip fracture; personal history of fracture related to mild-to-moderate trauma as an adult; poor health; chronic disease of the kidneys, gastrointestinal system, or lungs; sedentary lifestyle; and unhealthy lifestyle (tobacco smoke, excessive alcohol, or poor eating habits). The more risk factors you have, the more likely that your bone density will be low and the higher your risk for fracture will be. Since certain risk factors are not within your control, it's even more important to reduce or eliminate all of those that you can.

Secondary Osteoporosis

When bone loss occurs from another disease process or is due to a medication, it's called *secondary osteoporosis*. There are many genetic, endocrine, autoimmune, neurological, and allergic disorders that cause bone loss, as well as many medications.

DISEASES THAT CAN CAUSE SECONDARY OSTEOPOROSIS

Here's a list of some of the more common diseases that can cause secondary osteoporosis: adrenal gland insufficiency, ankylosing spondylitis, autoimmune disease, cancer, celiac disease, Crohn's disease, Cushing's disease, cystic fibrosis, diabetes, hyperparathyroidism, hyperthyroidism, inflammatory bowel disease, lung disease, multiple sclerosis, osteogenesis imperfecta, Parkinson's disease, and primary biliary cirrhosis.

MEDICATIONS ASSOCIATED WITH SECONDARY OSTEOPOROSIS

These medications are associated with secondary osteoporosis: glucocorticoids; excess thyroxine; antiseizure drugs, such as phenyton and phenobarbital; lithium; cytoxic chemotherapy (anticancer drugs); depot medroxyprogesterone acetate (Depo-Provera) birth control; heparin (long term); thiazolidinediones (e.g., Avandia, or rosiglitazone) for type 2 diabetes; proton pump inhibitors; and selective serotonin reuptake inhibitors (SSRIs) for depression and anxiety.

You may recognize one or two of these that you're currently using. Thyroid medications, for example, are commonly prescribed and can cause excessive bone loss if not monitored. Anticonvulsants interfere with calcium absorption, and proton pump inhibitors have recently been linked to osteoporosis. These and many other drugs can cause bone loss, so make sure to ask your doctor if any of the medications you are taking, or have taken in the past, are linked to an increased risk for fracture.

Glucocorticoids. Topping the list of bone-robbing drugs are the glucocorticoids, such as prednisone and cortisone. They are commonly used to treat inflammatory conditions such as rheumatoid arthritis, asthma, and systemic lupus erythematosus. These medications are so potent that 50 percent of patients taking them for over six months become osteoporotic. Even low-dose prednisone of 2.5 mg per day is known to increase fracture risk (Heffernan et al. 2006). If you are currently using a glucocorticoid, be sure to discuss this risk with your doctor. Bisphosphonate medications can be very beneficial for reducing the high fracture risk of glucocorticoid-induced osteoporosis.

Thiazolidinediones. Another commonly used group of medications linked to bone loss are the thiazolidinediones, such as Avandia (rosiglitazone) and Actos (pioglitazone hydrochloride), for the treatment of type 2 diabetes. These drugs are often prescribed with no mention of their potentially adverse side effect on bone. Diabetes is a serious disease and not taking these medications as prescribed could lead to serious problems. However, if you are diabetic, it may be possible for you and your doctor to reduce your need for thiazolidinediones by stabilizing your blood sugar through supplementary nutrition, diet, and lifestyle changes.

Proton pump inhibitors. Proton pump inhibitors (PPIs), such as Prilosec (omeprazole) and the "purple pill," Nexium (esomeprazole), are commonly prescribed for acid reflux or heartburn and the symptoms of gastroesophageal reflux disease (GERD). These medications not only cause bone loss from impaired calcium absorption, they also diminish levels of vitamins such as B_6 and B_{12}. Deficiency in B vitamins can lead to poor energy levels, weakness, and loss of balance—symptoms that put anyone with fragile bones at much greater risk for fracture. PPIs reduce *epigastric* (above the stomach) pain by depressing HCl (hydrochloric acid) production in the stomach. Stomach acids need to be strong to digest food, but they are caustic when refluxed upward into the esophagus.

By using a drug to reduce acid secretion, the symptoms of heartburn are averted. But the body's processes for digesting food and absorbing nutrients are impossible without stomach acidity. An article in the *Journal of the American Medical Association* cites a study linking PPIs to increased risk for hip fractures (Yang et al. 2006), which is not surprising considering their detrimental effects on digestion. With poor digestive capability, the absorption of important nutrients for bone health, such as calcium, zinc, magnesium, and the B vitamins, is compromised.

Although heartburn is often thought to result from excess acid production, more often it is caused by the opposite—too little acid secretion. *Hypochlorhydria*, or low gastric acid secretion, leads to poor digestion and to the *putrefaction* (rotting) of undigested foods in the stomach. Gases from these undigested or poorly digested foods cause bloating and force acidic juices up into the esophagus, where they cause pain and inflammation. Instead of reducing stomach acid secretion with a PPI, most people would benefit simply by eating more slowly, chewing their food thoroughly, adding vinegar to their meals when possible, and using over-the-counter digestive aids.

Note: Digestive aids such as betaine hydrochloride and pepsin should not be used if you have ulcers or regularly take medications, such as nonsteroidal anti-inflammatory drugs (NSAIDs) that are known to cause ulcers.

If you are experiencing GERD-like symptoms and your doctor has recommended a PPI for hyperacidity, you can confirm this diagnosis with a *Heidelberg test*. This involves swallowing a special vitamin-size pH-sensitive capsule that accurately measures your stomach's acidity. Before adopting PPIs to manage heartburn, ask your doctor to help you find a practitioner who will provide this testing. An easier alternative would be to take a tablespoon of apple cider vinegar with your meals or generously douse your salad with vinegar before meals. If you experience fewer heartburn symptoms, then your pain is due to hypo- not hyperchlorhydria. Next try some HCl and digestive enzymes; they'll probably prevent your heartburn and at the same time improve your bones through better digestion.

Thiazide diuretics. When discussing medications with your doctor, keep in mind that he or she may not be aware of every possible negative effect of the medications you may be taking. For example, thiazide diuretics are often prescribed to people with osteoporosis to reduce their loss of calcium through their urine. Although thiazides do have this effect, their role in reducing fractures is controversial (Cauley et al. 1993), and they actually increase urinary losses of vitamin B_6, magnesium, potassium, and zinc. Thiazides also have been linked to an increase in falls (Cauley, Salamone, and Lucas 1996), which are the number one cause of fractures in the elderly.

Because studies have shown that urine calcium can be reduced by vitamin K (Bügel 2003), potassium (He et al. 2005), and boron (Palacios 2006), why would anyone want to add a risk factor by taking a thiazide when it's probably not necessary? If your doctor determines that you have excess calcium in your urine, try this plan: Increase fruits and vegetables to eight to ten servings a day. Eliminate high-phosphorus cola drinks. Moderate your intake of red meats. Minimize your dairy intake (replace this calcium source with supplemental microcrystalline hydroxyapatite or calcium citrate/malate); and avoid caffeine. Supplement with vitamin K (1 to 5 mg/day), potassium bicarbonate (300 to 900 mg/day), magnesium (400 to 600 mg/day), and boron (10 mg/day).

EVALUATING YOUR FRACTURE RISK

Unfortunately, no one can ever really tell you your actual risk for breaking a bone. It's all a guessing game. But at least it can be a speculation based on facts. When evaluating your fracture risk, you must consider three variables: BMD, osteoporosis risk factors, and your chances of falling. Your fracture risk is estimated from a combination of those factors. The prime predictors for sustaining a fracture are your age and any history of breaking a bone as an adult. These two factors are even more important than your T score. Most fractures result from a fall. Muscular weakness and poor balance can turn an electrical cord or the turned-up edge of a rug into a hazard. That's why the major benefit of exercise as you age is not to add bone density, but to maintain strength, balance, and coordination, and thus decrease your chance of falling.

Quantity vs. Quality of Bone

Low bone quantity, as defined by your BMD T score, is a strong predictor of fracture, but it is not a measure of bone strength. Bone can have so much calcium and phosphorus bonded to its matrix that it becomes brittle. Therefore *bone strength* must be defined as a function of both its quantity and quality. Unfortunately, the medical establishment's current focus on DXA examinations, and their assessment of bone quantity as the single defining characteristic of bone strength, fail to acknowledge the quality of bone as of equal, or even greater, importance in resisting fracture.

Any mechanism that abnormally intensifies the remodeling process will quickly reduce bone's structural quality. As bone's microarchitecture deteriorates, its fragility increases as rapidly as a blight can overtake a forest. This loss of bone quality can happen fairly quickly and increase the risk for fracture, even when there is no noticeable reduction in the person's bone quantity as seen in his or her T score.

Chronic inflammation can cause osteoclasts to become aggressive scavengers of mineralized bone. Instead of digging shallow resorption pits that the osteoblasts can easily fill with new bone, inflammation-driven osteoclasts establish a huge number of basic multicellular units (BMUs) and excavate what look like deep miniature crevasses. Such intensive remodeling multiplies the risk of fracture even when BMD is not exceptionally low. This heightened state of remodeling transforms BMUs into tiny perforations similar to those in a notepad that make it easy to rip out a page. In the skeleton, these weakened zones accumulate microfractures that have the potential to "rip." Once started, localized rips lead to structural collapse and then to a catastrophic hip or vertebral fracture.

Overly exuberant remodeling is not the only factor that can degrade bone quality and increase fracture risk. Abnormal deterioration of bone collagen also can contribute to this acceleration of aging. Within the matrix, collagen fibers help to toughen bone and make it resistant to the bumps and jolts of daily life. However, when the collagen loses its suppleness, the bone stiffens and becomes brittle. If more mineral quantity is added with no attention paid to improving the quality of bone, stiffening is only accentuated and actually may increase the bone's fragility. We see this in older individuals who continue to fracture even when taking bisphosphonates to harden their bones.

And now we are starting to see more and more cases of low-trauma fractures of the *femoral shaft* (thigh bone) in women who have taken the bisphosphonate alendronate (Fosamax) for more than four years. This is increasing evidence that long-term use of bisphosphonates oversuppresses bone metabolism and creates a dangerous level of microdamage, which can eventually lead to catastrophic fractures (Neviaser et al. 2008).

The significance of bone quality for providing strength to bone can also be seen in diabetes. Type 1 diabetes is associated with low BMD and an increased risk for fracture. In type 2 diabetes, which is characterized by insulin resistance, there is also an increase in fracture risk, but, surprisingly, these patients have normal to even slightly increased levels of BMD. It's thought that in both types of diabetes, fracture risk increases, at least in part, due to a stiffening of the collagen and a loss of overall bone quality. The elevated blood glucose of a person with diabetes stimulates the formation of molecules called *advanced glycation end products* or AGEs. These troublesome molecules increase osteoclastic bone resorption and tightly bind to collagen fibers, acting like starch to stiffen bone and rob it of suppleness, and thus increase its fragility (Saito et al. 2006). This is a good example of the way that bones are part of a whole physiology—not separable structures like girders.

For these reasons your fracture risk cannot be based entirely on your T score. So begin thinking more in terms of bone quality and focus a little less on your BMD. Throughout this book you'll learn how to reduce your risk of fracture by improving the factors related to both quantity and quality. You will do this by first identifying therapeutic targets from your signs, symptoms, and lab tests, and then by implementing therapy to change those targets.

BIOCHEMICAL MARKERS OF BONE TURNOVER

Bone quantity and quality are compromised if there is too much resorption by the osteoclasts or not enough bone formation by the osteoblasts. The quantity of bone can be measured easily and fairly accurately through DXA testing, but there is only one way to directly evaluate bone's quality components: to bore a piece of bone tissue from the pelvis and analyze it under a microscope. But bone biopsies are painful and costly. Fortunately, there are now laboratory tests called *bone turnover markers* that can measure bone quality indirectly. This is done by measuring the degree to which bone turnover is occurring; that is, how aggressively the osteoclasts are eating bone, and the rate at which osteoblasts are building new bone.

Overly aggressive osteoclasts that destroy bone quality can be compared to a horde of carpenter ants that bore a maze of destructive tunnels through a tree trunk. Just as ants tend to burrow through the trunks of sick, elderly, weakened trees, osteoclasts become aggressive in physiologically weakened bodies. An infested tree looks strong from a distance, but up close its base reveals small piles of sawdust-like *frass* (insect excrement)—a telltale sign that the tree suffers from poor health and is slowly and silently being destroyed from within. The deep resorption pits of aggressive osteoclasts can have a similarly destructive effect on the quality of your skeleton. And just as with the infested tree, very few signs of excessive bone destruction can be spotted easily—at least not until we take a closer look.

By using specific bone turnover markers, called *resorption markers,* to assess the level of osteoclastic activity we can see not sawdust, but bone dust: small pieces of collagen released into the circulation and then excreted from the body in the urine. The amount of collagen detected is directly correlated to how much bone the osteoclasts are destroying.

Resorption Markers

Determining your rate of bone resorption is important for defining your fracture risk. Rapid bone loss indicates excessive osteoclastic activity and too many basic multicellular units. Remember the perforated paper analogy? That's what you want to avoid. When resorption markers are elevated, there is a higher risk for fracture no matter what your level of BMD (Garnero et al. 1996). Even if your bone density is not quite low enough to qualify for osteoporosis, an abnormal elevation in your resorption marker can indicate that you are at greater risk for fracturing (Greenspan and Luckey 2006).

There are three bone resorption markers that your doctor can order; however, he or she will need to order only one. The markers all look at the same resorption process, but each uses different technology. Specific to bone health, these biomarkers are the best therapeutic targets available. Use them. But the one your doctor chooses must be measured every several months or so. Examining the changes to your bone resorption process over time is the only way to assess your therapy's effectiveness.

Here's how it works: If your doctor orders a resorption marker test and your level is found to be abnormally elevated, this is your *therapeutic target marker.* Because you have not yet started treatment, it is considered your *pre-therapeutic baseline marker.* You now know that chronic inflammation can increase osteoclastic bone resorption, and in chapter 4 you will find out about several lab tests correlated to inflammation that, if found to be elevated, can be normalized by lifestyle changes and nutritional supplementation. By reducing these inflammatory markers, most likely there will also be a reduction of the bone resorption marker on subsequent testing. It is this serial testing that will enable you to determine your response to treatment.

If you have an elevated resorption marker, it *must* be reduced. I will show you ways to do this (such as reducing systemic inflammation) in later chapters. A drop in the level of a resorption marker indicates less osteoclastic activity, reduced bone loss, and lower fracture risk.

The three types of bone resorption tests are:

- **N-telopeptide (NTX).** This marker measures the small molecules of bone collagen being excreted through the urine. High levels of NTX are associated with rapid bone resorption and low bone mass in both men and women. By testing every several months, it's easy to monitor and determine the effectiveness of your nutritional therapy. Substantial drops in NTX indicate a reduction in bone loss and less risk for fracture.

- **C-telopeptide (CTX).** This is a similar marker to that of NTX, but CTX measures a different part of the collagen molecule. This marker can be tested from either a urine or blood sample.

- **Deoxypyridinoline (DPD).** This marker is tested, like NTX, by using a urine sample. Biological and analytical variability can be a problem with bone resorption markers, but measurements of DPD seem to be most consistent. Variability can be kept to a minimum if you make sure serial testing is always preformed through the same laboratory.

Caution: If you are currently using a bisphosphonate medication but have not had a pre-bisphosphonate baseline resorption test, the use of these markers as therapeutic targets for assessing the effectiveness of nutritional intervention will not be helpful.

Bone Formation Markers

The ability of osteoblasts to form bone can be measured clinically through three different tests—serum osteocalcin, serum bone-specific alkaline phosphatase, and serum P1NP. Unlike the resorption tests, each of these formation markers is typically used for a different situation.

OSTEOCALCIN

Osteocalcin is a protein produced by osteoblasts; it's important for activating the mineralization of bone. Therefore, it can be used as a biomarker for osteoblastic activity and bone formation. Note that determining whether your osteoblasts are forming enough bone can be especially helpful if your bone resorption marker (NTX, CTX, or DPD) is normal. Let's take an example: If you have osteoporosis and your bone resorption marker NTX is measured at 42 nmols (which is just about where it should be), then this would suggest that your low bone density may not be due to excessive resorption but to inadequate bone formation. Checking your osteocalcin level would be the next logical step. In all likelihood, it will read on the low side. Then your goal is to target osteocalcin and increase its levels on subsequent measurements.

However, osteocalcin can also register too high, especially during times of excessive bone remodeling. In this case, both your bone resorption marker and your osteocalcin would be elevated and your goal would be to reduce them both. To sum up, your primary goal when using a resorption marker like NTX as a therapeutic target is to reduce it, while your goal with the bone formation marker osteocalcin is to normalize it. In later chapters you will read about ways to do this. Whether your osteocalcin is high or low, vitamin K is necessary for its activation, so make sure your intake of this important vitamin is optimal.

BONE-SPECIFIC ALKALINE PHOSPHATASE

This test is essential for anyone taking a bisphosphonate medication for osteoporosis. *Bone-specific alkaline phosphatase* (bsALP) detects early signs of osteoblastic activity and is therefore useful for determining the oversuppression of bone resorption during bisphosphonate therapy (Kress et al. 1999). Remember, it's actually the osteoclasts that stimulate the osteoblasts to form bone. So if your osteoclastic activity has been oversuppressed by bisphosphonate medications, all the stages of your bone remodeling will be reduced, including bone formation by the osteoblasts. If you are currently taking a bisphosphonate, your doctor can monitor bsALP for oversuppression of bone remodeling. If your bsALP falls too low, he or she can reduce the dosage of your medication or even put you on a temporary drug vacation.

PINP.

If you are presently using or considering the use of teriparatide (Forteo), a daily injectable medication for very severe osteoporosis, you should talk to your doctor about the *PINP test*, which is the acronym for amino-terminal propeptide of type-1 procollagen. This test measures the amount of collagen in your blood serum and directly reflects the activity level of your osteoblasts (Melkko et al. 1996). Its primary use is for monitoring a person's response to teriparatide therapy (Eastell et al. 2006).

LOOKING AT YOUR SIGNS AND SYMPTOMS

When evaluating health we look for every clue we can find. You just read about laboratory biomarkers for assessing bone remodeling, and in later chapters you will learn about other, less specific, but nonetheless extremely helpful markers for monitoring bone health. But we can also use signs and symptoms for this same purpose. Just as your doctor looks for signs and inquires about symptoms related to secondary disease, you can look at your signs and symptoms related to nutritional deficiency and physiological dysfunction.

The signs and symptoms first discussed in chapter 1 are found below, but now their related deficiencies or dysfunctions have been added. These signs and symptoms are those most commonly presented by my patients with bone loss. My experience has been that when these are made better or more tolerable, patients' overall health improves and physiological pathways relevant to skeletal health benefit. Be sure to highlight or circle the signs and symptoms that pertain specifically to you.

GENERAL SIGNS AND SYMPTOMS AND POSSIBLE CAUSES

Fingernails. *Brittle:* general nutrient deficiency; digestion or malabsorption issues—need for amino acids, biotin (a B vitamin), calcium, zinc, and/or other minerals; can also be due to thyroid problems. *Flattening of nails with raised ridges or depressions:* anemia, iron deficiency, also seen in hemochromatosis (iron-overload genetic disease that causes bone loss) and in protein deficiency. *White streaks or spots on nails:* zinc. *Chronic soft tissue infection around nail:* zinc. *Pitted (psoriatic) nails:* vitamin D.

Hair. *Dry, brittle*—protein, biotin. *Thin, lifeless, low luster*—essential fatty acids, iodine. *Easily plucked*—protein.

Skin. *Bumpy skin on back of arms*—essential fatty acids, vitamin A. *Dry, scaly, flaking*—vitamin A, zinc. *Seborrhea in nasal folds along sides of nose to corners of mouth*—essential fatty acids. *Easily bruised, small areas of bleeding under the skin*—vitamin K or C, bioflavonoids. *Psoriasis, eczema, seborrhea, dandruff*—essential fatty acids, vitamin B_3, sulfur, zinc. *Dermatitis (inflammation as with eczema)*—zinc. *Hypersensitive skin*—magnesium.

Lips. *Cracks at edges of mouth*—B vitamins, especially riboflavin (B_2), iron, zinc.

Tongue. *Decreased taste or smell*—zinc. *Yellow coated*—poor digestion. *White coated*—yeast infection. *Painful, swollen, and reddened tongue*—B_2, B_{12}, folic acid.

Teeth. *Dental caries and premature tooth loss*—commonly seen in osteoporosis. *Periodontal disease (bleeding, swollen gums)*—vitamin D or C, bioflavonoids, riboflavin (B_2), folic acid, calcium.

Muscle. *Spasms*—magnesium, calcium, potassium. *Weakness*—vitamin D, protein.

Bone. *Tenderness of sternum or shins*—vitamin D, iodine. *Calcification of soft tissues (such as blood vessels and cartilage) seen on X-rays*—vitamin K.

This information was adapted from the *Textbook of Functional Medicine* (Jones and Quinn 2006).

GASTROINTESTINAL AND URINARY SIGNS AND SYMPTOMS, AND POSSIBLE CAUSES

Abdominal. *Bloating, prolonged fullness after eating*—need digestive enzymes and/or probiotics, lactose intolerance, abnormal gut flora. *Sensitivity to many foods*—food allergy, poor digestion.

Upper GI tract. *Belching*—need digestive enzymes and/or bile salts for fat digestion.

Lower GI tract. *Constipation*—magnesium, fiber, probiotics. *Copious gas*—poor digestion, food allergy, check for gluten intolerance, digestive enzymes. *Pale, foul-smelling stool*—need digestive enzymes, fiber, and probiotics. *Pale stool that floats in bowl water*—need bile acids. *Sensitive right lower abdominal area*—food allergy. *Diarrhea*—dysbiosis (overgrowth of abnormal bacteria in gut).

Urinary. *Frequent urination*—excess calcium excretion, food allergy.

INDICATIONS OF POOR SYSTEMIC HEALTH, TOXICITY, AND POSSIBLE CAUSES

Dark circles under eyes—food allergy, toxicity, poor digestion (need digestive enzymes). *Sensitivity along outside thighs*—overall toxicity. *Chronic morning stiffness*—food allergy, poor digestion (need digestive enzymes). *Frequent headaches*—food allergy, toxicity, (need poor digestion, need digestive enzymes). *Weight loss*—amino acids. *Depression, fatigue, anger*—general ill health, chronic inflammation, need full nutritional and emotional support.

Note: All signs and symptoms can be used only as potential indicators of deficiency or dysfunction. Physical signs and symptoms can result from many conditions; some of them serious and life threatening. It's important to consult your doctor about any sign or symptom that causes you concern. The signs, symptoms, and correlates to nutritional deficiency and physiological dysfunction listed above are not meant for diagnostic purposes. The information above should be used only as a guide and indicator for further testing.

Following are brief discussions of a few of the signs and symptoms listed above:

Fissures at corners of the mouth. An irritation or fissuring at the corners of the mouth, called *angular stomatitis*, is often seen in those with deficiencies of riboflavin, iron, or zinc. Nutrient-deficient-related stomatitis is often seen in those sensitive to the gluten protein found in wheat, barley, and rye, a condition called *celiac disease*.

White spots on fingernails. White spots on fingernails are linked to a deficiency of minerals, especially zinc. Though usually linked to immune health as well as to cellular growth and repair, zinc is also important for bone health. Its deficiency contributes to osteoporosis (Lowe, Fraser, and Jackson 2002). The white spots of zinc deficiency are often seen with malabsorption syndromes such as celiac disease.

Dandruff, scaly skin, bumps on back of arms. Essential fatty acids are integral components of every cell in your body, including bone cells. Fatty acid deficiencies contribute to chronic inflammation and to a loss of calcium through the urine—both of which lead to bone loss. Dandruff, scaly skin, and bumps on the back of the arms are classic signs of essential fatty acid deficiency.

Weight loss, depression, and fatigue. This triad of symptoms—weight loss, depression, and fatigue—is common in people with osteoporosis. These symptoms indicate a catabolic physiology and the need for intense nutritional support. (*Catabolism* is the destructive phase of metabolism in which complex substances are converted into simpler forms. Having a *catabolic physiology* means that the body is being broken down from its highly functional and complex form into one that is declining. See "Metabolism" in chapter 3.) None of these signs and symptoms is specific to osteoporosis, but all of them are linked to important aspects of your skeletal health.

LABORATORY TESTING

There are several laboratory tests that I consider the basic core in evaluating low bone density. They are the following:

- Comprehensive metabolic panel (CMP). A comprehensive metabolic panel is also referred to as a blood chemistry screen (SMAC). A CMP is a group of twelve to twenty tests used to screen the level of general health. These tests include an assessment of your electrolytes (sodium, potassium, chlorine, and carbon dioxide), kidney function (BUN and creatinine), liver function, bilirubin, alkaline phosphatase, and other assessments, such as albumin, calcium, cholesterol, triglycerides, glucose, lactic acid, phosphate, total serum protein, and uric acid.

- Complete blood count (CBC)

- Vitamin D [25(OH)D]

- Urine pH (morning)

- Urine calcium (either a calcium to creatinine ratio or a twenty-four-hour urine calcium test)

- Celiac profile (consisting of anti-tissue transglutaminase and antigliadin antibodies)

- Some form of bone resorption biomarker (NTX, CTX, or DPD).

These are just the bare-bones basic core for evaluating osteoporosis.

PUTTING IT ALL TOGETHER

Remember Ms. Hart from earlier in this chapter? She was my feisty, fifty-year-old patient whose second DXA exam had revealed osteoporosis. When Ms. Hart walked into my office she was very frustrated. "I don't understand it," she said. "I'm taking calcium, lots of it. How can I still be losing bone? What type of calcium *should* I be taking?" she asked. "My doctor wants to put me on a medication and I'm not sure I want to do that. Maybe it's not safe. Don't I have any other options? I feel so old, like I'm falling apart." And then Ms. Hart began to sob, "Where do I start? How can I get my bones strong again?"

Ms. Hart's frustration level, although high, wasn't unusual. With osteoporosis, it's difficult to know which way to turn. So, let's take a close look at Ms. Hart's questions and then walk through the assessment of her bone loss. Seeing how her bone loss was evaluated and treated, you'll have a much better idea of what to do for your own bone loss.

Choosing a Calcium Supplement

Ms. Hart's question about which calcium supplement to take is one I'm asked every day in my office. I suggest avoiding calcium carbonate and products containing oyster shell or dolomite as their major source of calcium. Some of these products are known to be contaminated with lead. Calcium carbonate from products like the antacid Tums is less absorbable than other forms of calcium. I usually recommend microcrystalline hydroxyapatite to my patients. It has the added benefit of containing natural growth factors for bone (Nugmanova et al. 2006).

Calcium citrate, dicalcium malate, and calcium bisglycinate chelate are also great sources for calcium supplementation. Take 1,200 to 1,500 mg of calcium a day. Make sure the supplement you choose is guaranteed free from harmful additives and toxins. Most importantly, never take calcium without also including a good supplemental source of magnesium. These two minerals work together. Their ratio in your diet should be at least two to one (calcium to magnesium).

Unless you are taking calcium carbonate, the benefit of taking one form of calcium over another is slight. Your choice probably won't make much difference to your overall fracture risk. In a study done in Australia, researchers showed that taking calcium carbonate (1,200 mg/day) reduced the risk for fracture in women from 16 percent to 10 percent over a five-year period (Prince et al. 2004). That's impressive for such a poor source of calcium. What's important is to take your calcium—and your magnesium.

Are Osteoporosis Medications Safe?

Ms. Hart's question concerning the safety of osteoporosis medications is important. In recent years increasing concerns about the medications used to treat osteoporosis have surfaced. For example, hormone replacement therapy (HRT) was the mainstay of osteoporosis treatment until the Women's Health Initiative study was halted prematurely in 2002. This study revealed that HRT with synthetic estrogen and progestin increased the risk of breast cancer, heart disease, stroke, and blood clots (Anderson et al. 2004).

Over the past decade, the use of bisphosphonate therapy has replaced HRT as the osteoporosis treatment of choice. But these new medications carry their own risks. Bisphosphonates have the potential to increase fractures later in life, and according to Dr. Anthony Pogrel, an oral surgeon from the University of California Medical Center in San Francisco, they can even cause *osteonecrosis of the jaw* (ONJ) in young adults from the oversuppression of bone remodeling (2004). This serious condition of exposed jawbone can lead to infection and unrelenting pain and disfigurement, and is very resistant to treatment.

Ms. Hart's concerns are very real. Osteoporosis medications should be used only when absolutely necessary. Nutritional support, on the other hand, should be the primary approach to bone loss and it should be accompanied by pharmaceutical intervention only when fracture risk is moderately elevated. For Ms. Hart, other than her T scores we had no information concerning her fracture risk, so a prescription for medication would have been premature.

Ms. Hart's Examination

Ms. Hart appeared to be quite healthy, but a lengthy consultation and examination proved fruitful. Other than her low body weight of 124 pounds, history of depression, and being postmenopausal, Ms. Hart had no other known risk factors for osteoporosis. The following lists summarize important findings related to her risk factors and her physical signs and symptoms.

Bone Status Date	Bone Status Date
Osteopenia: 3/14/2001	Osteoporosis: 2/20/2006
Spine T score: -2.3	Spine T score: -2.8
Hip T score: -1.4	Hip T score : -1.6

Risk Factors	Signs
Low body weight (124 pounds)	Abdominal bloating Excessive gas
History of depression	White spots on fingernails
Postmenopausal	Small crack in skin at edge of her mouth (cheilosis)

Symptoms

Depression

Feelings of anger

Ms. Hart's complaints of abdominal bloating and gas were of primary concern. These symptoms prompted my suspicion of a possible malabsorption disorder. Moreover, the white spots on her fingernails and the *cheilosis* (cracks around her mouth) were signs of a nutritional deficiency that often accompanies poor absorption. My first thoughts were that her osteoporosis might have been caused by a gluten sensitivity that had resulted in celiac disease. Being sensitive to gluten can damage the small intestine so severely that its ability to absorb nutrients becomes disrupted. Gluten sensitivity also activates inflammatory mechanisms. Together, malabsorption and inflammation lead to bone loss.

In addition, Ms. Hart's history of depression and anger, coupled with her substantial bone loss, made me suspect that she might be harboring a high level of inflammation. However, other than the two concerns, celiac disease and chronic inflammation, nothing else from her examination gave me any clues to the cause of her bone loss. But these were enough. Look at the information below for the results of the lab tests I used to evaluate Ms. Hart's bone loss.

MS. HART'S LAB TESTS AND RESULTS

- *Comprehensive metabolic panel* (CMP): All tests were normal.

- *Complete blood count* (CBC): All tests were normal.

- *Vitamin D* [25(OH)D]: 27 ng/ml; insufficient. Sufficient levels are considered 35 to 80 ng/ml.

- *Urine pH* (morning): Average of 5.6 on serial testing; abnormally low. Normal pH averages between 6.0 and 8.0.

- *Urine calcium* (24-hour sample): 322 mg/day; abnormally high. Upper limit for women is 250 mg/day.

- *Celiac profile* (anti-tissue transglutaminase [tTGA] and antigliadin antibodies). *Results for tTGA*: 15.0 EU/ml. Normal reference range is less than 20. When tTGA is above 20, it's considered positive for celiac disease. *Results for antigliadin antibodies*: IgG—31.3 EU/ml (normal reference range is less than 28). IgA—24.1 EU/ml (normal reference range is less than 23). Antigliadin antibodies, when elevated, indicate a sensitivity to the gluten protein in grains.

- *NTX* (bone resorption marker): 130 nmolBCE/mmol; high. Abnormal if above 70 nmolBCE/mmol.

- *Homocysteine*: 11 nmol/L; high. Normal is below 8 nmol/L.

- *High-sensitivity C-reactive protein*: 1.7 mg/L; high. Abnormal if greater than 1.0 mg/L.

Ms. Hart's Assessment

Ms. Hart's urine NTX test indicated that she was losing bone rapidly. This troubled me. High NTX is a major risk factor for fractures. So reducing her NTX level became our top priority. Her metabolic panel and blood count were both normal, which helped to rule out major organ involvement, but her vitamin D—the most important vitamin for bone health—was low. Vitamin D aids in the intestinal absorption of calcium, and Ms. Hart certainly needed supplementation. But even though her tests indicated that she had inadequate stores of vitamin D, I didn't think this was the cause for her elevated NTX. Her low vitamin D levels might reduce her ability to absorb calcium and make bone—but it wouldn't cause her to lose bone. Something else was causing that.

One common finding in people with osteoporosis is an excessive loss of calcium in the urine. So I wasn't surprised when Ms. Hart's twenty-four-hour urine calcium test came back elevated. She was losing lots of calcium. This often occurs when a person is acidic, and Ms. Hart's first morning urine pH averaged a very acidic 5.4. But once again, even though this was an important finding, and even though we needed to increase her pH and reduce her calcium loss, this was not the cause of Ms. Hart's high NTX.

When assessing patients with bone loss, one of the first things I look for is some type of disruption in their ability to absorb nutrients. There are several malabsorption syndromes that can cause bone loss, but they are usually accompanied by loose, foul-smelling stools and a high level of fat (along with gas) in the stool that causes the stool to float and creates a greasy film on the water in the toilet bowl. Ms. Hart didn't have any of these signs or symptoms, but she did have abdominal bloating and excessive gas. Celiac testing of tTGA ruled out celiac disease. So what was the cause of Ms. Hart's elevated NTX?

The final two tests I ordered for Ms. Hart were homocysteine and C-reactive protein. These are biomarkers of inflammation. In addition to her osteoporosis, her symptoms of depression and signs of anger added to my concern that she might be burning up on the inside.

Homocysteine is an acid produced in the body from the breakdown of the amino acid L-methionine. An elevated level of homocysteine is commonly seen in people with chronic inflammation and, traditionally, has been linked to an increased risk for heart disease. Its detrimental effects are also linked to osteoporosis (McLean et al. 2004), and in a study at the University of Bergen in Norway, researchers lead by Dr. Clara Gram Gjesdal (2007) showed that the higher the blood levels of homocysteine, the greater the fracture risk.

High sensitivity C-reactive protein (hs-CRP) is produced by the liver in response to inflammation. Similar to homocysteine, hs-CRP is also seen as a risk factor for heart disease. But we now know that elevated hs-CRP is also linked to bone loss and an increased risk for fracture. One study (Stewart et al. 2008) reported that hostility and depression act together to raise chronic inflammation and are correlated with elevated levels of hs-CRP.

I felt that the hs-CRP was clearly a diagnostic test to be ordered because Ms. Hart had struggled with depression for years and was extremely emotional. Not surprisingly, both homocysteine and hs-CRP came back positive. Finally, we'd found two good reasons for her elevated NTX. Ms. Hart was burning up from inflammation and now we had several therapeutic targets to focus upon. This was the beginning of successfully managing Ms. Hart's bone loss.

Ms. Hart's Treatment Plan

Ms. Hart had four signs we could use as therapeutic targets: bloating, gas, white spots on her nails, and cheilosis. By taking her off gluten all of these resolved quickly. Although she did not test positive for celiac disease, Ms. Hart's tests indicated she was somewhat sensitive to gluten. To be safe, we eliminated all gluten from her diet and, not surprisingly, her abdominal bloating and excessive gas quickly disappeared. To me, this was a good sign that even though she did not technically have celiac disease, her gluten-caused abdominal distress was probably contributing to her loss of bone. Over the next several months, Ms. Hart's cheilosis resolved and the white spots on her nails disappeared with the help of 25 mg per day of supplemental zinc.

Ms. Hart's symptoms of depression and frustration were, of course, more complicated and difficult to use as therapeutic targets. For her general health I recommended a good multivitamin-mineral supplement, a calcium-magnesium product, whey protein, and an amino acid blend to help build her tissues.

Her laboratory tests provided six biomarkers to work with as therapeutic targets. For her low vitamin D, Ms. Hart began taking 2,000 IU of vitamin D_3 each day. This would help bring her vitamin D blood levels to above 35 ng/ml. When recommending vitamin D to patients, I also suggest taking vitamin K, which helps to increase bone density and reduce fracture risk. Vitamin K is found in two major forms, K_1 and K_2. A recent study (Knapen, Schurgers, and Vermeer 2007) showed an increase in the bone content and strength of the hip bone with the use of vitamin K_2. In this study, 45 mg per day of vitamin K_2 in the MK-4 form was used, but the authors suggest that the longer-acting vitamin K_2 MK-7 may be a better choice and the amount needed could then be reduced. (MK-n simply stands for menaquinone-n, the type of vitamin K produced by bacteria and its specific biochemical version)For my patients I recommend a combination product of vitamin K that includes K_1 and K_2 in both the MK-4 and MK-7 forms. This is what I recommended for Ms. Hart.

Ms. Hart's excessive loss of calcium through her urine was because her body was extremely acidic. By recommending that she substantially increase fruits and vegetables in her diet, reduce sugar intake, supplement with vitamin K, boron (10 mg/day), and potassium bicarbonate (600 mg/day) before bedtime, her calcium loss was reduced and her urine pH increased from 5.4 to an average of 6.4.

Ms. Hart's homocysteine and C-reactive protein levels were invaluable therapeutic targets. Her homocysteine was reduced by supplementing her diet with vitamins B_2, B_6, B_{12}, and folic acid. Her C-reactive protein dropped from 1.7 mg/L to 0.9 mg/L by adding fish oil, flaxseed, vitamin C, alpha-lipoic acid, N-acetyl cysteine, and milk thistle, all of which are important antioxidants and help to reduce inflammation. I also recommended that she take curcumin, a biologically active compound extracted from the spice turmeric. Curcumin is well-known for its excellent anti-inflammatory activity and it can stimulate the activity of vitamin D (Jurutka et al. 2007) and improve BMD.

The final therapeutic target, and probably the most telling for improved bone health, was dealt with easily. I knew that by reducing Ms. Hart's inflammation, the aggressiveness of her osteoclastic activity (and her bone loss) would decrease. This was reflected in the reduction of her resorption marker. Over the next year Ms. Hart's NTX dropped from 130 to 55. At this point I knew that we had saved Ms. Hart from the ravages of osteoporosis.

The following text summarizes Ms. Hart's therapeutic targets and her treatments.

MS. HART'S THERAPEUTIC TARGETS AND THERAPEUTIC PLANS

- *Osteopenia*: Spine T score -2.3; hip T score -1.4. DXA date 3/14/2001.
  Treatment: No therapeutic action was taken by her doctor at that time.

- *Osteoporosis*: Spine T score -2.8; hip T score -1.6. DXA date 2/20/2006.
  Treatment: Basic bone support in the form of calcium (microcrystalline hydroxyapatite complex), magnesium, vitamins C, D, B_{12}, and K, folic acid, boron, trace amounts of strontium, zinc, manganese, copper, and silicon. Basic nutritional support in the form of a multivitamin complex (with vitamin A from mixed carotenoids, not retinol), whey protein powder (20 g/day), and fish oil or krill oil.

MS. HART'S RISK FACTORS AND TREATMENT PLANS

- *Risk*: Low body weight (124 pounds on 2/25/2006).
  Plan: Gain muscle mass through nutrition and exercise.

- *Risk*: History of depression.
  Plan: Improve nutrition.

- *Risk*: Postmenopausal (one year; last period at age forty-nine).

MS. HART'S SIGNS, SYMPTOMS, AND TREATMENT PLANS

- *Abdominal bloating, excessive gas*: Eliminate gluten from diet.

- *White spots on fingernails*: Zinc.

- *Small crack at edge of mouth (cheilosis)*: B vitamins, zinc (Ms. Hart was not iron deficient).

- *Depression*: Improve diet, plus emotional and psychological support.

- *Frustration and anger*: Reduce chronic inflammation through diet changes plus fish oil, vitamin C, alpha-lipoic acid, N-acetyl cysteine, and milk thistle. Add emotional support.

MS. HART'S LAB TESTS AND THERAPEUTIC PLANS

- *Low vitamin D* (3/15/2006): Supplement vitamin D_3 (2,000 IU/day), vitamin K_1 (1 mg/day), and vitamin K_2 (MK-4, 1 mg/day, and MK-7, 50 mcg/day).

- *Low urine pH* (3/15 to 3/19): Increase fruits and vegetables, decrease red meat.

- *High urine calcium* (3/15/2006): Increase fruits and vegetables; supplement with vitamin K (as above), boron (10 mg/day), and potassium bicarbonate (600 mg/day).

- *High antigliadin antibodies* (3/15/2006): Eliminate gluten.

- *High NTX* (3/15/2006): Reduce inflammation. Increase consumption of oily fish such as salmon; add hemp oil or flaxseed to diet; reduce red meat unless range-fed; add omega-9 fats, such as olive oil, almonds, and avocados; eliminate hydrogenated or partially hydrogenated oils; and supplement with fish oil, vitamin C, alpha-lipoic acid, N-acetyl cysteine, milk thistle, and curcumin.

MS. HART'S ADDITIONAL TESTS AND THERAPEUTIC PLANS

- *High homocysteine* (3/24/2006): Supplement vitamins B_2 (25 mg/day), B_6 (50 mg/day), B_{12} (500 mcg/day), and folate (use active form of 5-methyltetrahydrofolate, 400 mcg/day).

- *High levels of high sensitivity C-reactive protein* (3/24/2006): Reduce inflammation by supplementing with fish oil (3 g/day), flaxseed, vitamin C (1 g/day), alpha-lipoic acid (300 mg/day with biotin), N-acetyl cysteine (2,000 mg/day), milk thistle (400 mg/day), and curcumin (400 mg/day).

EXERCISE 2.1: THERAPEUTIC TARGETS

Take all the time you need to complete the following exercise. When complete, it will be a summary of your current bone status (osteopenia or osteoporosis), risk factors, and the designated therapeutic targets derived from all of your signs, symptoms, and laboratory tests. This is a great way to compile all your skeletal health information in one place.

1. Go back to the section "Looking at Your Signs and Symptoms," and look at the signs and symptoms that you circled or highlighted.

2. Now pick up your journal and take some blank pages to write down the headings for the chart you will now make for your own signs and symptoms. On the first page of your journal, write the headings "Bone Status," "Date," and "Treatment Plan." On the second page, write the headings "Risk Factors" and "Indication/Treatment Plan." On the third page, write Signs and Symptoms and Treatment Plan, and on the final page, write Lab Tests, Date, and Treatment Plan.

3. Then go to the signs and symptoms that you marked or highlighted and copy them under the appropriate headings in your journal. Also, be sure to write down the results of any lab tests that you may have already obtained. Highlight any abnormal test results and write them down. Make sure to include the date that the test was taken. If you have repeat testing done, you can add to this list later.

4. This is a great way to compile all of your skeletal health information in one place. When you complete it, it will be a summary of your current bone status (osteoporosis or osteopenia), risk factors, and the designated therapeutic targets from all of your signs, symptoms, and laboratory tests.

By now I hope that you're beginning to see the immense potential that signs, symptoms, and biomarkers can provide in the diagnostic and therapeutic approach to osteoporosis. Gone are the days of "take this or that supplement and hope for the best." Also gone are the days of taking medication for osteoporosis without first obtaining an evaluation for fracture risk, and the days of ignoring nutrition as a primary therapeutic approach to bone loss.

SAMPLE JOURNAL PAGES FOR EXERCISE 2.1

Bone Status	Date	Treatment Plan

Page 1

Risk Factors		Treatment Plan

Page 2

Signs and Symptoms		Treatment Plan

Page 3

Lab Tests	Date	Treatment Plan

Page 4

CHAPTER THREE

How Healthy, Soft Tissues Foster Healthy, Strong Bones

Sight a tree in the distance. Its silhouette, composed of a leafy, energy-gathering top and a woody, supportive trunk, is pleasing in its balanced proportions. Its shape denotes health and evolutionary success for the species. What is important for this analogy is to realize that the harder structures—the branches and trunk—grow only in response to the demands of the softer structures—the leaves, blossoms, and seeds. The more foliage the tree holds, the stronger its trunk must grow. Robust growth, additional weight, and the potential for greater stresses brought by winds require stronger support. This is similar to the relationship between your own soft tissues and the supportive structure of your bones. As leaves, blossoms, and seeds send signals to woody trunks, so too do muscles, fat, and soft organs send signals to bone. Messages for skeletal strength are conveyed during times of soft-tissue growth, and the need for conservation of energy is signaled during times of stress, disease, or dwindling resources.

THE CONNECTION BETWEEN SOFT TISSUE AND BONE HEALTH

Remember from the last chapter that low body weight was listed as a major risk factor for osteoporosis? This makes sense because the lower your body weight, the less bone strength is needed for support. The commonly accepted myth that your skeleton automatically strengthens when you ingest more calcium is far too simplistic—soft-tissue growth is required as the stimulus for bone formation. Ingesting a full complement of nutrients, even with extra helpings of calcium, will not strengthen your bones unless a signal is first sent by your soft tissues to indicate this physiological need. The place to start then is to put some meat on your bones.

When I speak of soft tissues, I'm predominately referring to fat and lean muscle tissue. Each of these tissues affects bone mineral density (BMD) differently. Fat cells maintain BMD by producing estrogen and another hormone called leptin. Muscle tissue affects your BMD by involving your skeleton in strenuous activity. Fat and muscle are both important, but research has shown that muscle mass is more critical for maintaining bone density (Wang et al. 2005). In fact, one study (Travison et al. 2008) suggests that maintaining muscle mass is the best strategy you can take to maintain your bone health as you age. A short discussion about metabolism is now in order.

How Metabolism Works

Metabolism is the entire complex set of ongoing chemical reactions in our bodies that are necessary for survival. Regulated by enzymes and hormones, these chemical reactions allow you to grow, repair tissues, convert food into energy, stay warm, and a zillion other important functions. Metabolism is comprised of two separate activities that occur simultaneously. One is anabolism, or constructive metabolism, and the other is catabolism, or destructive metabolism. Both were discussed briefly in chapter 1.

Anabolism takes place when your body takes small components, such as amino acids from protein-rich food, and actively laces them together to form specialized tissues, such as muscles, nerves, organs, connective tissues, and bone. *Catabolism* is the opposite process. This occurs when your body takes components from digested food and tears them apart to extract chemical energy for use as fuel. For optimal health, these two processes—anabolism and catabolism—must be kept in perfect balance.

In a chronic disease like osteoporosis, catabolism dominates. This state is brought about by a body so out of kilter and so desperate for energy that it goes beyond attacking mere digested food; it turns to breaking down its own tissues. Instead of maintaining mineral-rich bone, the mineral-deficient catabolic body, in its effort to maintain normal blood pH levels, is constantly mining its own skeleton for the alkaline minerals essential for sustaining life.

A loss of muscle mass and tone can indicate an inflamed catabolic physiology. Catabolism not only melts away muscle, it also gives it a loose, spongy, and lifeless feel. When muscle tissue wasting is severe, it's called *sarcopenia*, and it is commonly seen in people with osteoporosis.

EXERCISE 3.1: Tissue Poke

When I say "soft tissue," remember that I'm referring to muscle and fat tissue. First, pinch yourself—not just your skin, but the full amount of tissue covering your bones. Then, gently poke yourself in your sides, buttocks, arms, and thighs. Use all your fingers. When you have finished poking yourself, rate each statement below by circling a number from 1 to 5.

1. My tissues feel spongy like dough.

I don't feel like this at all.   1 2 3 4 5   This describes what I am feeling.

2. My muscles feel loose and floppy.

I don't feel like this at all.   1 2 3 4 5   This describes what I am feeling.

3. My muscles lack firmness when I flex them.

I don't feel like this at all.   1 2 3 4 5   This describes what I am feeling.

4. My tissues have less bulk to them than they did five or ten years ago.

I don't feel like this at all.   1 2 3 4 5   This describes what I am feeling.

5. My bones seem to be sticking out of my skin.

I don't feel like this at all.   1 2 3 4 5   This describes what I am feeling.

6. My buttock tissue sags and doesn't feel firm and rounded.

I don't feel like this at all.   1 2 3 4 5   This describes what I am feeling.

7. I have slumped posture and I feel my back is weak and doesn't hold me up straight.

I don't feel like this at all.   1 2 3 4 5   This describes what
                                                                I am feeling.

8. My abdomen protrudes.

I don't feel like this at all.   1 2 3 4 5   This describes what
                                                                I am feeling.

Total _____

Scoring: Now add up your score. If you circled mostly 4s and 5s, then your tissues may not be sending strengthening messages to your bones—even if you took your calcium today. A score of 20 or greater may indicate that you have sarcopenia. If this is the case, you need to make it your mission to enhance the health of your soft tissues so that they will start to signal your bones to get stronger. This means consuming a healthy anabolic-promoting diet, eliminating the factors that interfere with tissue growth, and increasing weight-bearing and resistance-training exercise.

PROMOTING SOFT TISSUE HEALTH FOR STRONGER BONES

How do you get your soft tissues to send the correct messages to your bone? Read on and you will find out how to do that.

Provide Optimal Nutrient Quality and Adequate Quantity

Your nutritional goal should be to make yourself as strong and healthy as possible—at every meal. Bone health cannot be achieved just by taking supplements. In fact, excessive supplementation with isolated nutrients has the potential for deleterious effects to your health. For example, a recent study (Bolland et al. 2008) found that the rise in *serum calcium*, that is, calcium circulating in the blood, from calcium supplementation may accelerate vascular calcification and increase the risk for heart attack.

Your body requires a constant balanced intake of nutritionally stimulating food; supplementation should be used only to normalize deficits and to rectify abnormalities in your body's functioning. Haphazard or unbalanced supplementation creates problems. For example, a high intake of calcium can create relative deficiencies of other nutrients, such as magnesium and vitamins D and K, which are often already at insufficient levels. It's important to establish a supplemental regime that is both therapeutically balanced and not potentially harmful.

In addition, by focusing on isolated nutrients instead of diet, you may miss out on biologically active compounds and the cumulative effects of nutrient interactions obtained through foods. For example, *isoflavones* (estrogen-like compounds found in soybean products) and *flavonoids* (plant pigments with antioxidant, anti-inflammatory, and anticancer properties, plentiful in oranges, blueberries, and prunes) are known to have bone-building qualities. The citrus flavonoids diosmetin and quercetin, found in orange pulp, and other flavonoids like myricetin in walnuts and kaempferol in broccoli and grapefruit are all known to have anti-inflammatory effects, as well as the ability to increase osteoblastic activity (Hsu and Kuo 2008). Beverages such as green tea, bicarbonate-rich mineral water, and acacia juice also have beneficial effects on bone.

DIETARY RECOMMENDATIONS FOR GOOD BONE HEALTH

There is no exact bone-healthy diet. Today, most people know that fruits and vegetables, especially vegetables, should be at the top of their nutritious foods list. You also need a good amount of protein, but obviously not an excessive amount. One interesting, and often disturbing, fact about my osteoporosis patients is that many of them seem obsessed with the foods they should or should not consume. They have become so focused on their diet that all of their joy in eating has been lost. This is in no way beneficial.

Eating for optimal skeletal health doesn't have to be complicated. Certainly, questioning every bite that you ingest is counterproductive. That said, it is still important to understand that if you have osteoporosis, you are in a nutritionally deficient hole. A good, healthy diet, one that is adequate for someone in good health, may not be adequate for you. You can climb out of the hole you're in only by eating well, supplementing your diet with specific nutrients, not worrying excessively about small details, and making sure that you are enjoying life. You don't have to cook anything special. Just follow these general recommendations and you'll be fine.

Don't eat on the run. Low-stress dining is important. When you eat too fast, you don't absorb nutrients efficiently.

Eat four to five times a day. It's best not to go for long periods without eating. Each time you go for five or more hours without eating, your adrenal glands have to pump out more of the hormone *cortisol* to maintain your blood glucose levels. This is very stressful for these glands. Moreover, constantly elevated cortisol levels reduce osteoblast activity, lower BMD, and increase fracture risk. Eat frequently, but only to satiation.

Try to eat as much fresh, unprocessed, and organic food as possible. This is common sense, but you also want to avoid foods with additives, preservatives, and pesticides. Processed foods add a toxic load to your body. Plus, they usually lack antioxidants and other nutrients.

Eat five to nine servings of fruits and vegetables each day. Most fruits and vegetables are alkaline and help to reduce the adverse, bone-robbing effects of the typical acidic Western diet of meat and potatoes.

Reduce the grains. A diet high in grains like pasta, cereal, and bread causes your body to become overly acidic. Grains are also high in inflammation-producing omega-6 fatty acids and low in the anti-inflammatory omega-3s. Try to limit grains to only one or two servings a day. Eat vegetables instead.

Eat protein. Protein is very important for the construction of bone matrix. Eat wild-caught seafood, naturally raised poultry, and lean, range-fed beef. Since the amino acid lysine is essential for bone health, make sure you are eating enough quality protein. Not only does lysine help to absorb and conserve calcium, it is also important for forming bone collagen. Because it is mostly found in meat, poultry, fish, and eggs, vegetarians are often lysine deficient and would do well to supplement their diet with 500 mg per day.

Consume omega-3 fats. Salmon, mackerel, herring, and tuna are all high in protein and omega-3 fats, which help to reduce inflammation. Hemp seed oil and flaxseeds (soak them in water for best results) are a great sources of omega-3s in the form of alpha-linolenic acid. It's best to use flaxseeds instead of the oil because flaxseeds also contain lignans, which are important for skeletal health. (*Lignans* are found predominantly in the hull of flaxseeds and are antioxidants that have estrogen-like properties.)

Consume omega-9 fats. *Omega-9s* are monounsaturated fats found in high amounts in olives, almonds, hazelnuts, and avocados. These fats help to reduce the pro-inflammatory effects of saturated fats. Omega-9 fats also help to increase the "good" cholesterol HDL, and reduce the "bad" cholesterol LDL. Omega-9 fats contain polyphenols, which act as antioxidants. These help to reduce inflammation and have been shown to reduce the risk for osteoporosis. There is truth to the saying that an apple—or perhaps I should say five olives—a day keeps the doctor away.

Go easy on the dairy products. If you do eat dairy, make sure you aren't sensitive to the protein casein, and that you are able to digest its lactose sugar. (See chapter 5.)

Avoid hydrogenated or partially hydrogenated oils. These oils are found in just about all of the processed foods displayed on grocery store shelves. Hydrogenated oils dramatically increase the inflammation in your body. When you cook, use butter, extra-virgin olive oil, or, my favorite, virgin coconut oil, which contains MCT (medium-chain triglyceride) fatty acids.

Limit refined carbohydrates. Sugar not only robs you of important minerals, it also increases the release of insulin from your pancreas and lowers levels of an important hormone called insulin-like growth factor 1 (IGF-1). As you will see later in this chapter, IGF-1 is very important for bone health. When cutting back on sugar (sucrose), try to avoid fructose as a substitute, and instead use maple syrup, honey, xylitol, stevia, or agave—but be moderate in your use of any of these. *Xylitol*, also called "birch sugar" because it is made from birch trees, is the only sweetener that has been shown to have a beneficial effect on bone. One study (Mattila, Svanberg, and Knuuttila 2001) found that xylitol reversed bone loss in animals, possibly by promoting calcium absorption from the gut.

Go easy on the salt. High-salt diets are linked to low bone density, especially when a person has chronic low-level metabolic acidosis (Frings-Meuthen, Baecker, and Heer 2008).

Keep vitamin A intake in check. Levels of vitamin A intake above 10,000 IU per day have been linked to low bone density (Feskanich et al. 2002). Vitamin A is important to health and has been added to a lot of products, so it's wise to read labels. Keep your total vitamin A intake at 5,000 to 8,000 IU per day with no more than 5,000 IU per day of *retinol* (the active form of vitamin A).

Eat Soy. It may be good for your bones but... According to a literature review (Setchell and Lydeking-Olsen 2003), the isoflavones daidzein and genistein, found in soy, have been shown to reduce bone loss in animal studies, but the results of human studies are still problematic. The reason for this may stem from the observation that these isoflavones may first need to be activated by the gut's microflora before they are able to have an anabolic effect on bone (Mathey et al. 2007). Therefore, if your gut health and microbial balance are poor, activation of soy isoflavones will be compromised and their potential to benefit bone will be minimized. But even if research suggests that soy increases bone density in humans, there will still be the question of whether or not it is able to actually reduce the incidence of fractures (Morabito et al. 2003). Until these issues are resolved, soy should be consumed only in moderation.

Soy is also a common allergen, so be cautious if you have any digestive complaints. Also, if you have an underactive thyroid or a hormone-sensitive cancer, your soy consumption should be kept to a minimum.

Take bone-building phytoestrogens. Plant products with weak estrogenic activity, such as isoflavones and lignans, are called *phytoestrogens*. In the form of lignans they can be found in nuts, vegetables, and especially freshly ground flaxseeds. Flax is important to add to your diet because it is high in both the anti-inflammatory omega-3 fatty acids and the bone-building lignans. If you are a woman and have osteoporosis, you should include flaxseeds in your diet. There have been concerns about men using flax oil because of a possible connection with prostate cancer. Because of this I recommend that men use only flaxseed.

Drink mineral water. Mineral waters from Europe are high in bicarbonate (make sure they have at least 500 mg/L), which helps to alkalinize your body. This is good for your bones.

Eat oranges, broccoli, and onions. These are great foods for bone health. They provide bioactive compounds that have been shown to increase bone density.

Eat soups. Making fresh soups with lots of vegetables is easy and provides wholesome nourishment. When you're cooking with meat, be sure to include the bone.

My favorite foods for bone health. Sardines, broccoli, almonds, and prunes.

KEY NUTRIENTS FOR BONE HEALTH

The appendix contains important information on specific bone nutrients. It includes a description of each nutrient, deficiency signs and symptoms, related laboratory tests, helpful correlated laboratory tests, dietary sources, and supplement recommendations. Most of the tests I've listed are usually available through your doctor. As you will see, I haven't included tests for every nutrient because they may not be commercially available or their accuracy is questionable. I haven't listed many tests that have recently become available through specialty labs. These tests, such as those for amino acids, fatty acids, organic acids, toxic elements, and mineral levels of red blood cells can all be very helpful, but they are beyond the scope of this book. When you create your bone-healthy diet, refer to the appendix for all of this very important information.

AVOID THE BONE ROBBERS

What you don't put into your body is almost as important as what you do. If you want good bones, you have to limit your alcohol intake, stop smoking, not salt your food excessively, go easy on the sugar, and not consume cola beverages. By eliminating the unhealthy aspects of your lifestyle and diet, you will have better bones.

Be aware that certain foods tend to increase inflammation in the body. The major culprits are corn-fed beef, saturated fats, hydrogenated and partially hydrogenated fats, sugar, and sunflower, corn, and safflower oils. Use these foods as infrequently as possible.

Ensure Good Digestion

Nutrients don't just show up in your bones. You need to jump-start the process of anabolic repair through good digestion.

BOOST DIGESTIVE HYDROCHLORIC ACID AND ENZYMES

Look back at the signs and symptoms in chapter 1 and chapter 2. If you marked abdominal bloating, gas, or belching as symptoms, you may not be receiving all the nutrients from your diet that you thought you were getting. These symptoms indicate that you are having difficulty digesting your food. This difficulty may be contributing to your loss of bone density.

Abdominal symptoms from poor digestion can be caused by inadequate production of the stomach's hydrochloric acid (HCl) or digestive enzymes. As we get older, our ability to produce HCl decreases. You may have noticed an increase in your digestive-related symptoms. Digestive problems are often the root cause of osteoporosis. Their negative impact ripples throughout the body, getting worse, not better, as we age. Frequently, the first response after being diagnosed with bone loss is to reach for a bottle of calcium. Ironically, if you have poor digestion, adding alkaline calcium to your stomach only serves to further neutralize, or buffer, your already ailing level of digestive acids. This further compromises digestion and creates even more intestinal complaints.

If you are experiencing digestive symptoms such as bloating, belching, and excess gas, consider taking an oral digestive aid. You can purchase various blends containing HCl and the digestive enzymes pepsin, pancreatin, bile, and others. Your health care provider may be able to help you determine which digestive aids will be most beneficial for you.

When taking betaine hydrochloric acid with meals, start by taking one tablet (750 mg) with your first meal, two with your second meal of similar size, and so on. Observe whether your digestive symptoms improve after meals. If you notice a warm sensation in your stomach, decrease the number of tablets at your next meal. You may need to vary your intake of HCl depending on the size of the meal. I would recommend not taking more than five tablets per meal. Over time, you should be able to reduce the number of tablets. That's because your stomach—and you—are getting healthier.

GOOD DIGESTION LEADS TO HORMONE ACTIVATION

Every time you eat, your digestive enzymes break down the food into absorbable molecules and stimulate the release of several important hormones (Reid, Cornish, and Baldock 2006). Growth hormone, ghrelin, leptin, insulin, insulin-like growth factor 1, and others make it possible for your body to utilize absorbed nutrients. These hormones are the factors that kick-start the anabolic repair process. They initiate a turning of the catabolic tide.

Growth hormone. Also referred to as somatotropin, growth hormone is produced by the anterior pituitary gland in the brain. It is a powerful stimulator of growth and cell reproduction. It stimulates production of cartilage and bone, and is especially important during child development for the growth and lengthening of bones in the arms and legs. But the need for growth hormone doesn't stop with the onset of adulthood or, for that matter, in your older years. It has very powerful antiaging effects and keeps your bones healthy by stimulating calcium absorption, bone production, and mineralization.

Because growth hormone is anabolic, we want to stimulate its production and release. Sleep, exercise, dietary protein, and estrogen all promote the release of growth hormone. On the other hand, refined carbohydrates and emotional stress reduce its production.

Ghrelin. Released by the stomach, ghrelin acts to stimulate the secretion of growth hormone in anticipation of the influx of nutrients. Ghrelin is a natural appetite stimulant, and its blood levels rise as mealtime approaches. If you don't eat, ghrelin notifies you with hunger pangs. Elevated levels of ghrelin also stimulate the brain to release growth hormone for anabolic repair. If you still don't eat, growth hormone starts looking around for other sources of nutritional building blocks. It sends out signals to break down "expendable" tissues, of which bone is a primary target. In the order of essentials for life, bone is not at the top of the list. In fact, if you remember, part of the skeleton's job description is to act as a mineral reservoir, and to release those minerals during times of need. If you don't eat regularly, you're creating a catabolic situation for your bones that is best avoided.

Leptin. This hormone is a product of fat cells and is involved in appetite regulation. As body weight increases, engorged fat cells release more leptin. This rise in the hormone's blood levels acts to block hunger receptors in the brain, thus reducing the desire to eat. This, of course, affects nutrient intake and skeletal health. Leptin also takes a more direct role in the regulation of bone remodeling. It does so in two ways and with two opposing results. Centrally, from within the brain, nerve impulses flow out through the body to the bone cells in the skeleton when leptin blood levels rise. As this leptin-induced nerve activity increases, it reduces the bone-building activity of the osteoblasts and therefore limits bone formation (Pogoda et al. 2006).

Peripherally, from the soft tissues and inside the bone marrow, the leptin released by fat cells directly stimulates receptor sites on billions of osteoblasts in the skeleton and causes a completely opposite effect. Leptin's direct stimulation of osteoblasts increases their bone-forming activity and blocks their release of RANKL (Holloway et al. 2002). You may remember from chapter 1 that the signaling molecule RANKL ordinarily activates osteoclastic bone resorption, but when leptin levels rise, RANKL release is curtailed and the osteoclasts become less active. This dual action of increasing osteoblast bone formation and reducing osteoclast bone resorption makes the direct action of leptin upon bone cells *osteogenic*, or bone building.

Leptin's combined effects, through both its central and peripheral influence on appetite control and bone remodeling, make this hormone vital to skeletal health. What we learn from observing the actions of leptin is that it is important to maintain a healthy body weight—enough fat to produce normal levels of the hormone leptin, but not so much fat that health is undermined in other ways.

Insulin. The hormone insulin is released from the pancreas in response to eating. Today, almost everyone is familiar with insulin's connection to diabetes. When you eat sweet foods, the sugars stimulate the release of insulin, which then transports glucose into your cells for energy. People with diabetes do not have the insulin necessary for this glucose transport, and therefore the amount of glucose within their blood rises. The longer glucose remains at an abnormally elevated level, the faster the person's health retreats.

For that reason, insulin is important for soft-tissue growth, and as you already may suspect, insulin receptors have been found on bone cells. Insulin stimulates osteoblasts to increase bone formation (Cornish, Callon, and Reid 1996), and although too much insulin is a sign of disease, normal levels are important for skeletal health.

Insulin-like growth factor 1 (IGF-1). This growth factor, along with its binding proteins, act to increase muscle mass and strengthen your bones. As its name implies, it is similar to insulin in its molecular composition, and the biological effects of insulin and IGF-1 do overlap. When you don't eat, insulin is not secreted; that's also true for IGF-1. Released from the liver in response to growth hormone, IGF-1 is the most powerful anabolic agent in the body. IGF-1 is also produced locally within the bone marrow, where it stimulates the osteoblasts to build bone.

IGF-1 is so important for bone health that I want you to make it your mantra. Repeat "IGF-1, IGF-1, IGF-1." It's been estimated that IGF-1 influences at least one-third of the factors involved in bone growth (Rosen et al. 2005), and it is not unusual to see low levels of IGF-1 in people with osteoporosis. Low IGF-1 also leads to the muscle wasting of sarcopenia. Go back to exercise 3.1 above. What was your score? Anything above 20 would raise suspicions of insufficient IGF-1. Its anabolic effects are so important that in a study of 350 elderly Swedish women, IGF-1 showed a stronger association to BMD than did vitamin D (Salminen et al. 2007).

Unfortunately, as we age, our bone cells have reduced ability to respond to IGF-1 stimulation (Cao et al. 2007). By ensuring adequate intake of essential fatty acids (as found in fish oil) you will help to maintain healthy cell membranes and receptor sites for important molecules like IGF-1. This will enhance your bone cells' ability to respond to the dwindling anabolic effects of IGF-1.

How can you increase your IGF-1? Eat lots of protein. In a randomized, controlled trial published in the *Annals of Internal Medicine*, patients with hip fractures who were able to increase their IGF-1 reduced their bone loss in just one year simply by increasing their protein intake (Schürch et al. 1998). If your doctor has tested you for IGF-1 and it is low, try supplementing your diet with the following. They have all been shown to increase IGF-1: whey protein (20 mg/day); milk basic protein (whey's basic protein fraction); conjugated linoleic acid (CLA); colostrum (the fluid in a mother's first milk, in this case from bovine sources, which stimulates the immune system); an amino acid blend (5 to 10 g/day; L-glutamine, L-arginine, L-lysine, L-ornithine, and glycine are especially important); dehydroepiandrosterone (DHEA) (25 to 50 mg/day); and zinc (25 mg/day). Note: If you have been diagnosed with hormone-sensitive breast cancer or any other hormone-sensitive disorder, taking DHEA is not recommended.

Promote Bone Renewal by Encouraging Healthy Body pH

Of your skeleton's three major functions—structural support, vital organ protection, and as a reservoir for alkaline mineral reserves—it is the last that is intimately connected to the loss of bone density. Your arterial blood pH must be maintained at approximately 7.4; even small changes in this measurement can be life threatening. Acidic ions, continuously produced in your body from normal biological activity, are buffered by the dietary intake of alkaline minerals. If your production of acidic ions is higher than your intake of potassium, magnesium, and calcium, then the minerals within your bones are tapped for use elsewhere in your body. This condition, called *chronic low-level metabolic acidosis,* leads to bone loss.

CHRONIC LOW-LEVEL METABOLIC ACIDOSIS

Metabolic acidosis can result from a diet high in salt and processed foods or excessive protein intake, and from prolonged, intense exercise, aging, ill health, airway disease, emotional stress, and menopause. But the biggest contributor to an acidic physiology is a phosphate-rich Western diet, which is high in sulfur-containing animal and grain protein, and low in alkaline fruits and vegetables. When your body is acidic, you lose more calcium through your urine, and consequently, your bone's osteoclastic activity accelerates. According to research conducted at University College in London, low body pH also causes your osteoblasts to stop making bone (Andrea Brandao-Burch 2003). It also lowers your IGF-1 levels (Jandziszak et al. 1998). By alkalinizing your body, you will increase IGF-1, reduce urine calcium loss, and balance the remodeling process, which maintains the health of your skeleton.

TESTING YOUR BODY pH

The only accurate method for analyzing body pH is through arterial blood. Arterial puncture is a more painful and potentially dangerous procedure than routine venous puncture and requires a special laboratory procedure. A less accurate but still valuable method of measuring body pH is through testing urine. Measuring the pH of your first morning urine will give you a good general perspective on your body's overall acid-alkaline balance. If your urine pH is consistently low, your body chemistry is acidic. To do this measurement, you will need litmus paper with gradations of 0.2 or 0.3, spanning a pH of at least 5.5 to 8.0 (a good source is Micro Essential Laboratory, www.microessentiallab.com.) Simply tear off a short strip of the litmus paper and let a small amount of urine flow onto it. Compare the strip's color to the chart included in the package. Ideally, your pH should be above 6.6. If it is consistently below 6.0 during repeat testing, you are most likely in a catabolic state of low-level metabolic acidosis. This is not good.

EXERCISE 3.2:   Morning Urine pH

Check your first morning urine pH for seven consecutive days. After the seventh day, average your readings and jot down your score. In your journal keep a record of your daily pH and weekly averages. In addition to urine pH, there are other test results that can indicate low-level metabolic acidosis. Your doctor will be able to assess the following tests and determine if their overall trend indicates metabolic acidosis:

- Excess calcium in your urine (*hypercalciuria*)

- Low-normal blood carbon dioxide (test on the CMP)

- Low-normal blood phosphorous (test on the CMP)

- Elevated $1,25(OH)_2$ vitamin D (the active form of vitamin D)

- Low IGF-1

- Mild low-functioning thyroid (mild hypothyroidism)

IMPROVING BODY ACID-ALKALINE BALANCE

Reducing excessive protein intake (cheese, especially hard cheese, meat, and grain products) and increasing your consumption of fruits and vegetables will bring the pH of your body into a better balance. Fruits such as berries, mangoes, cantaloupe, honeydew, and watermelon and vegetables such as broccoli, bok choy, cabbage, cauliflower, kale, onions, and asparagus are particularly good for this. Make sure that your salt intake is not excessive. Processed foods are very high in salt and should be avoided. A recent study (Frings-Meuthen, Baecker, and Heer 2008) demonstrated that a high salt intake contributes to low-level metabolic acidosis and increases urine calcium excretion and osteoclastic bone resorption.

If your urine pH continues to be less than 6.0, try taking two to three capsules (600 to 900 mg) of potassium bicarbonate or potassium citrate, 250 mg of magnesium, and 1 gram of taurine (an amino acid that helps regulate cell fluids) before going to bed at night. One study (Jehle et al. 2005) showed that neutralizing acidity with potassium citrate can increase bone density.

Reduce Oxidative Stress

Oxidative damage from free radicals is a major contributing cause of all degenerative diseases, including osteoporosis. We need oxygen to live, but there are metabolic consequences to this need. When molecules interact with oxygen, free radicals called *reactive oxygen species*, or ROS, are formed. Excessive oxidation and the formation of ROS can damage your cells. If there are more ROS in your body than you're capable of neutralizing, this is referred to as *oxidative stress*, and it results in cellular damage. The more ROS that go unneutralized, the more oxidative stress results, and the more your tissues will be damaged.

Most people think that free radicals come only from pollution in their environment. And it's true that cigarette smoke, excessive alcohol intake, industrial wastes, exhaust fumes, and even bacterial, viral, and fungal infections are huge sources of ROS free radicals and oxidative stress. But the production of ROS and oxidative stress also can come from within your own body, as the by-products of metabolic reactions within your soft tissues.

Before we can derive energy from food, it must first be digested and absorbed as small molecules through the gut lining. These molecules—amino acids from proteins, fatty acids from fats, and simple sugars from polysaccharides—are then transported into our cells, where oxygen is used to extract their energy. It's the job of the *mitochondria*, specialized *organelles* (functional units) within our cells, to extract this energy, but ROS are produced as by-products.

This ROS production is normal, even necessary, for your survival. But, in general, the healthier you are, the fewer the number of ROS your mitochondria will spew out as they extract energy for cellular activity, such as muscle contractions. When health deteriorates, an excess of ROS-induced oxidative stress occurs, and the end result is disease. Premature aging, cancer, heart disease, Alzheimer's, and osteoporosis are the consequences. To regulate ROS production, your soft tissues have developed protective mechanisms, using antioxidants, to keep you healthy.

Antioxidants can be enzyme molecules produced in your body or compounds that you ingest from food. In both cases, they act as free radical "scavengers." These scavengers protect you from damage by binding to ROS, inactivating them, and thus reducing oxidative stress. The healthier your soft tissues, the more they can produce protective antioxidant enzymes. The more antioxidant-rich fruits and vegetables you eat, the more effective you are at reducing the harmful effects of ROS.

For years, it was thought that estrogen deficiency was the primary cause for osteoporosis in women. Today we know that estrogen-related bone loss is much more complicated than that. When laboratory animals are deficient in estrogen, it has been shown that they accumulate ROS within their bone marrow. These free radicals are the actual cause of the animals losing bone density (Grassi et al. 2005). This may be the reason why some women lose BMD excessively at menopause and others don't. A woman who enters menopause (a time of increased ROS production) with an already elevated production of ROS from high oxidative stress will experience greater bone loss than if she had no preexisting oxidative stress. Grassi et al. (2005) demonstrated that ROS production and bone loss can be reduced with antioxidants such as N-acetyl cysteine. Antioxidants are so important for bone health that, in an article from the *Journal of Clinical Investigation,* the authors concluded that supplementation is important for all women with low estrogen (Lean et al. 2003).

HOW DO YOU KNOW IF YOUR BODY IS PRODUCING TOO MUCH ROS?

It is possible to identify excessive ROS production and the need for supplemental antioxidants through two laboratory tests. Both biomarkers can be used as therapeutic targets for antioxidant therapy if they are found to be elevated. The first test is a measure of serum lipid peroxides. When these oxidized particles of fat are found to be elevated, that indicates your body is becoming rancid from oxidation. Fortunately, you can take antioxidants such as vitamins C and E to prevent this rancidity.

The other test for excess ROS is 8-hydroxy-2-deoxyguanosine or 8OH2dG. This urine biomarker measures the amount of oxidative damage occurring within the DNA of your cells. Knowing whether you have excessive oxidation is crucial. As you'll see in chapter 4, the same oxidative process that damages lipids and DNA also prevents you from building bone.

HOW TO REDUCE ROS

To reduce ROS, don't smoke. Don't drink excessive quantities of alcohol. Reduce your stress. And don't overexercise—especially not next to a smoggy freeway. These activities all increase oxidative stress and your overall production of ROS.

Foods important for their antioxidant properties are berries, citrus fruits, leafy green vegetables, and, my favorite, prunes. Grapefruits are not only high in vitamins and rich in antioxidants, they also contain bioactive compounds helpful for building bone. A study from Texas A&M University found that grapefruit reduces ROS and improves bone quality in rats (Deyhim et al. 2006). But a note of caution: If you are currently taking medications, grapefruit can interfere with the way your body reacts to them. The consumption of grapefruit with any medication is usually contraindicated. Check this with your doctor before consuming grapefruit.

Vitamins C and E, alpha-lipoic acid, and N-acetyl cysteine are just a few of the many antioxidants available for reducing oxidative stress and ROS. That said, if your diet is high in fruits and vegetables, you wouldn't want to take excess antioxidant supplementation. There has been some concern that excessive antioxidant intake may have the potential for harm. Indeed, ingesting too many antioxidants can lead to pro-oxidant activity, which can be an antecedent of disease. A delicate intake balance must be maintained. Ask your doctor about serum lipid peroxide and 8OH2dG testing. When your body is deficient in antioxidants, supplementation can be essential for reducing bone loss.

Here is a short list of foods and nutrients that provide antioxidant activity: citrus fruits, such as oranges and lemons; fruits, such as watermelon, which is high in lycopene; vegetables, such as tomatoes, which are high in lycopene; prunes; vitamins C, E, and beta-carotene; and the minerals, selenium, copper, zinc, and manganese. Other supplements, such as N-acetyl cysteine, alpha-lipoic acid, ubiquinone (coenzyme Q10), resveratrol, and quercetin are also useful for reducing bone loss.

Stimulate Bone Formation Through Exercise

Exercise can be like a heaping spoonful of good medicine. A consistent regimen of weight-bearing exercise will improve bone health, increase muscle strength and coordination, and reduce your fracture risk. Being active not only helps sweep the cobwebs away by improving circulation and reducing systemic inflammation, it also sends the final spark that ignites bone renewal. Osteocytes are constantly sensing the mechanical strains your bones experience every time you move. If an area of bone is weakened, osteocytes send signals to the osteoclasts and osteoblasts to begin the process of remodeling for bone fortification. But if you're not physically active, there is no mechanical strain, and therefore no signals are sent.

To signal bone formation, you should engage in two primary types of exercise on a regular basis: weight-bearing exercise and strength or resistance training. Try to get a minimum of fifteen to thirty minutes of exercise, three to four days a week. If you're over forty or have any cardiovascular risks, such as high blood pressure or elevated cholesterol, you should talk with your doctor before beginning an exercise program. He or she may want to set certain limits for you regarding the level of exertion, the amount of weight-bearing exercise you can handle, and the best type of exercise you should do for your body. For example, bending forward or lifting weights overhead can put a heavy load on your spinal vertebrae. If your bone density is extremely low, this can overload your spine and cause a compression fracture.

So use good judgment and caution when exercising. But also, if you're able, do your best at pursuing an exercise program. If you've been cleared by your doctor, get to a gym, go out into the woods, or just move to music played in your living room. You were designed to be active, and movement will help you heal.

WEIGHT-BEARING EXERCISE

Weight-bearing exercise includes walking, jogging, hiking, tai chi, dancing, aerobics, yard work, tennis, stair-climbing, bowling—anything that has your body moving against the resistance of gravity helps to stimulate bone formation. But there are limits. The time in your life to have built bone was when you were an adolescent or a young adult. Adulthood is more the time for bone conservation. When you are older, weight-bearing exercise should be done to maintain bone density, not necessarily to gain it. You want to do enough exercise to tell your bones that they're needed, but not so much that you risk breaking one.

STRENGTH TRAINING

Muscle strength and bone strength are like twin brothers—they always stick together. If one gets sick, both suffer. For this reason, if you want to have stronger bones, you must exercise to get stronger muscles. One of the best ways to do this is through strength training, or what is often referred to as resistance exercise. *Strength training* involves moving your body against some form of resistance. This can include the use of free weights (dumbbells), weight machines, elastic resistance bands, or simply resisting your own weight, such as with abdominal crunches, wall push-ups, or squats. The great thing about exercise, even resistance training, is that it doesn't require fancy equipment. You can lift soup cans in your kitchen and receive great benefit. The main thing is to get into an exercise routine and stick to it.

If you're over the age of thirty, you're going to lose an average of 5 percent of your muscle mass each decade older you get. This only gets worse after the age of sixty-five, and that's the time when you need your muscles the most. Engaging in regular strength training to gain muscle mass not only helps you gain bone (or at least limits its loss), but by improving your muscle strength and coordination you will prevent falls, which are the leading cause of hip fractures. So get out there and do something. Exercise makes you feel better. Have fun. Of course, if you have a heart condition, ask your doctor first. That only makes sense.

Low-Magnitude, High-Frequency Vibration Platforms

If you are incapacitated or have bone density that is so low you cannot participate in weight-bearing exercise, there is another alternative available to you. Small vibration platforms have been developed that actually help to maintain your bone density. The mechanical strain that helps maintain bone density is not caused only by the large concussive forces of weight-bearing exercise. Dr. Clinton Rubin and colleagues from the State University of New York at Stony Brook, Department of Biomedical Engineering, have shown that the small-amplitude microstrains from muscular contractions may be of equal importance to bone health (2001).

Just five microstrains of mechanical stimuli (that which is produced by the contraction of a muscle) are enough to stimulate cells to produce bone. In an effort to mimic these small microstrains of muscular activity, Dr. Rubin has developed vibration platforms designed to build bone density.

The platforms emit up-and-down vibrations at a very low magnitude of 0.3 g-force (g for the earth's gravitational field) and of high frequency of 30 Hz. The mechanical signals produced from these vibrations are similar to those created by muscle contractions. Simply by standing on one of these vibrating platforms, anabolic signals are sent throughout the skeleton to build bone. In a study of seventy postmenopausal women, Dr. Rubin and colleagues (2004) showed that just twenty minutes a day on a platform can stop bone loss. Vibration platforms, therefore, are an excellent alternative form of exercise, especially if you are incapacitated or have suffered from previous fractures and cannot engage in weight-bearing exercise.

A note of caution when selecting a vibration platform: You don't want one that acts like the paint shakers found in hardware stores. There are several companies that sell these types of machines, and some of them vibrate too much. More vibration is not better and can actually cause harm. If you're considering the purchase of a vibration platform, make sure that it *oscillates* (vibrates) vertically, and be sure that the vibrations are approximately 0.3 g in magnitude and 30 Hz in frequency.

BODY MASS INDEX

Having healthy bones takes more than just having healthy soft tissue—you also need to have the right amount of it. Calculating your body mass index (BMI) is a great way to determine whether you are over- or underweight and prone to chronic disease. For osteoporosis, it's being underweight that we find to be most problematical. But you already knew that low body weight is a risk factor for osteoporosis. Dr. Ian Reid, professor of medicine and endocrinology from the University of Auckland, New Zealand, has clearly demonstrated that a person's soft-tissue mass reflects the level of his or her bone density (2002). That is, the lower your BMI, the more likely it is that your bones are being broken down faster than they're being built (Revilla et al. 1997).

EXERCISE 3.3:   Calculate Your Body Mass Index

You can calculate your own BMI simply by using the formula below. Then see what your score means by looking at the scoring information directly below that.

703 × (your weight in pounds ÷ [your height in inches × your height in inches]) = BMI

Go ahead. Do it. The calculation is done in this way: Take your weight in pounds and divide that weight by your height in inches times your height in inches. Multiply that number by 703, and that will give you your BMI.

703 × (_____ pounds ÷ _____ inches × _____ inches) = _____ BMI

BMI scoring: Below 18.5 is underweight. Between 18.5 and 24.9 is normal. Between 25 and 29.9 is overweight. 30 and above is obese.

If your BMI is below 18.5, you now have another therapeutic target. Your goal is to improve this number by just one-half point over the next six months. This will happen if you reduce muscle-wasting that results from your body being acidic, eat alkaline fruits and vegetables and monitor your first morning urine pH, and supplement with 20g per day of whey protein. Also get sufficient exercise. Let's see what can happen with your BMD if you increase your BMI.

CHAPTER FOUR

Chronic Systemic Inflammation and the Conflagration of Bone

Remember that wilderness trek you embarked on in chapter 3? Unfortunately, it has turned into a bit of a temporary disaster. Some careless hikers ahead of you had a guide who failed to properly manage their campfire. After they broke camp, hidden embers burst into flame, and now you are faced with a raging forest fire. Osteoporosis is similar to that campfire. The silent smoldering of chronic low-level inflammation that can lead to bone loss may be hiding beneath your skin like concealed embers. In many cases, this silent inflammation can ambush your skeletal health by fueling excessive bone resorption and limiting bone formation.

Not only does inflammation cause bone loss, it also can set the stage for other diseases. Heart disease, diabetes, Alzheimer's, depression, and even cancer all share a common unifying factor with osteoporosis: chronic inflammation. Even when age and shared risk factors are removed from the equation, there is still a clear relationship between osteoporosis and heart disease (Farhat et al. 2007). As you'll see, reducing inflammation is just as important for healthy bone as dousing the last embers of a campfire is for the health of a forest.

INFLAMMATION

Inflammation is your body's response to potentially harmful stimuli. Whether the threat comes from invading pathogens (viruses and bacteria), physical trauma, or chemical irritants, your body defends itself with a complex immune response of first isolating the invader, then destroying it, and, finally, healing from it. Your defenses begin at your skin's surface and extend to the mucous membranes of your respiratory, urogenital, and gastrointestinal tracts. If and when foreign molecules, referred to as *antigens*, breach these physical barriers, your immune system responds with an immediate inflammatory defense.

Acute Inflammation

Acute inflammation is your body's short-term response to infection or injury. Blood vessels swell, releasing fluids and white blood cells (WBCs) into the affected area. This is the source of the swelling, heat, redness,

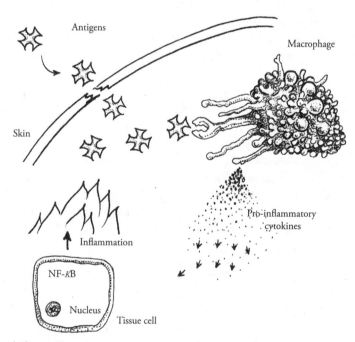

FIGURE 4-1: The innate immune response.

and pain that are the classic signs and symptoms of inflammation. Special WBCs, called *macrophages*, release signaling cytokines as they mount their attack on the foreign antigens. These *pro-inflammatory cytokines* signal the activation of *NF-κB* (nuclear factor-kappa B), a special protein found within the interior of every cell in your body. NF-*κ*B is like a matchstick waiting to be struck in order to ignite inflammation (see figure 4-1). Once activated, NF-*κ*B commands the cell's nucleus to turn on hundreds of inflammatory-inducing genes within its DNA. During the initial phases of defense, macrophages by the millions devour and destroy antigens. This is referred to as the *innate immune response*. If the invasion is a minor one, the macrophages subdue the threat right then and there.

But if the assault is more substantial and the macrophages are unable to contain the infection, a second system of defense is called in to do battle. The macrophages, along with another type of WBC called *dendritic cells*, summon the T cells for extra help. *T cells* are the commanding generals of all WBCs. They orchestrate this second, more powerful and specialized defense system, called the *adaptive immune response* (see figure 4-2). This second response is an aggressive process that can

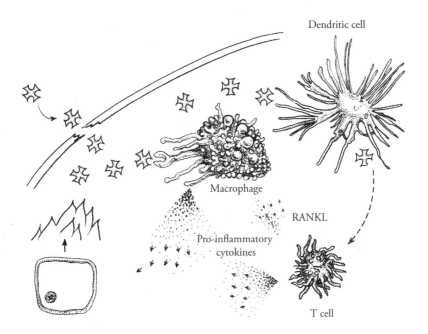

FIGURE 4-2: The adaptive immune response.

turn up the inflammatory fires of NF-κB. The T cells summon even more macrophages and dendritic cells by releasing pro-inflammatory cytokines and yet another molecule: RANKL. (As you'll remember from chapter 1, RANKL is also involved in activating osteoclasts during bone remodeling.)

CELLS OF THE IMMUNE SYSTEM

What follows is a brief description of the three most important WBCs—macrophages, dendritic cells, and T cells—all involved in the interactions between our immune and skeletal systems. Together, if and when inflammation turns chronic, these cells play key roles in the disrupting, or uncoupling, of the coupled interactions between osteoclasts and osteoblasts during bone's remodeling process. It is no coincidence that all three cells are born within bone's marrow.

Macrophages. These huge defense cells migrate from bone marrow by way of the bloodstream. They take up sentinel positions in the various tissues of the body. Macrophages will devour just about anything harmful that gets in their way, and then they signal T cells to activate the release of NF-κB for the inflammatory response.

Dendritic cells. These cells capture pathogens, rip them to shreds, and deliver their pieces to T cells for processing during the activation of the adaptive immune response.

T cells. These ultraspecialized cells command the adaptive immune response. From the bone marrow where they were made, immature T cells travel to the thymus gland (thus the "T" in T cell), where they mature. From the thymus gland, T cells travel to other parts of your body where they lie in wait within lymph nodes until they are needed.

Chronic Systemic Inflammation

Chronic systemic inflammation is an insidious, pathological condition that brews chronic disease. Once established, chronic inflammation's destructive forces burn deep into every tissue and organ system of the body. It evolves slowly, takes years to develop, and unfortunately, sometimes it takes years to extinguish.

Your body depends on just the right amount of inflammation from its immune system. Too little and pathogens may take over. Too much firepower and the immune system backfires, damaging your body. When activated, NF-KB normally stimulates the genes of inflammation for only an hour or so. The response disappears quickly when it's no longer needed. But if pro-inflammatory cytokines are persistently expressed by your immune cells for weeks, months, or even years, the immune system gets confused and becomes untethered from its control mechanisms. It swings grossly out of balance and its matchsticks (NF-KB) are perpetually being struck and lit. This is exactly what can happen in osteoporosis.

The adaptive immune response has two arms of defense. These arms are defined by the immune-mediating actions of two types of *helper T cells*, or *Th* cells, produced in the thymus gland. When viruses or bacteria burrow into your cells, the first arm, called *Th1* (Th for T cell helper), defends you by calling in the WBCs through the heavy release of pro-inflammatory cytokines. When invading pathogens infiltrate throughout your body attacking cells from every angle, the second arm, referred to as *Th2*, responds by sending out antibodies to identify and neutralize the intruders. This two-armed response has evolved over millions of years, and when used equally, each arm complements the other in a healthy and balanced immune response. But your life has been very different from that of your ancestors.

Today, you might present challenges to your immune system that it may not be prepared to cope with. Antibiotics, immunizations, toxins, antibacterial soap, and even your diet have changed the way your immune system reacts. Nowadays, it's not uncommon for a person's adaptive immune response to be lopsided and have one arm that is grossly dominant. It's as if you were lifting weights using only one arm and neglecting the other. After only a few weeks of working out in this manner you would become lopsided. When only one arm of your adaptive immune response is exercised, it begins to pump out high levels of cytokines specific to that arm's response. If Th1 becomes the dominant arm and it's not kept in check by Th2, the predominance of pro-inflammatory cytokines accentuates the activation of NF-KB, which then leads to uncontrolled inflammation.

T cells are aroused by more than bacteria and viruses. Toxins, free radicals, irritating foods, bacterial overgrowth, and even oxidized molecules of fat, glucose, and protein can arouse T cells and stimulate the release of RANKL in an unbalanced, predominately Th1 response (see figure 4-3). Over time, such irritants become the tinder for chronic systemic inflammation.

Chronic inflammation retains some of the same characteristics found in the acute inflammatory response. Both responses use the same pro-inflammatory cytokines and RANKL as signaling mechanisms, and both activate macrophages, dendritic cells, and T cells. But the classic signs of acute inflammation—swelling, heat, redness, and pain—are suspiciously absent. A chronic response is ineffective; it's like an army of soldiers racing around with torches but without specific orders to follow. A chronic inflammatory response is worthless. It's incapable of fighting off antigens and just smolders away, inflaming helpless tissues.

Cytokines

Cytokines are the small signaling proteins used by WBCs to affect the immune response and trigger inflammation. Some cytokines turn on inflammation (pro-inflammatory); others turn it off (anti-inflammatory). When inflammation is chronic, the cytokines that turn it on are excessively abundant and those that turn it off are scarce or ineffective.

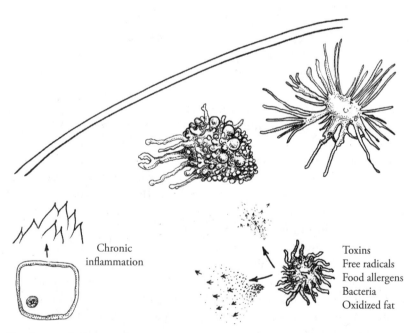

Chronic inflammation

Toxins
Free radicals
Food allergens
Bacteria
Oxidized fat

FIGURE 4-3: A predominant Th1 immune response eventually leads to chronic inflammation.

PRO-INFLAMMATORY CYTOKINES

In our study of the immune and skeletal remodeling systems, we are mainly concerned with three pro-inflammatory cytokines: interleukin-1 (IL-1), interleukin-6 (IL-6), and tumor necrosis factor (TNF). The term interleukin means "messenger between leukocytes," which are the WBCs. All three of these cytokines are produced by the immune cells to promote mechanisms involved in the inflammatory response.

RANKL

There are many other cytokines than the pro-inflammatory types mentioned above; however, we will concentrate on just one of them. That cytokine is RANKL, receptor activator for nuclear factor-*K*appa B ligand (RANKL). This protein is a signaling cytokine that activates NF-κB and the inflammatory response. T cells release RANKL to summon macrophages and dendritic cells to an infected area during the adaptive immune response.

NEXUS OF THE SKELETAL AND IMMUNE SYSTEMS

Overlapping biochemical pathways functionally connect the immune and skeletal systems. Not only do pro-inflammatory cytokines and RANKL play critical roles in inflammation, they also have primary functions to carry out in the remodeling of bone. This overlap in signaling is the cornerstone that links the immune system to bone loss.

When the immune system is out of balance and the Th1 arm of the adaptive immune response dominates, the outcome is destructive cross talk between the two systems that ends in disease. When the immune system is unbalanced, cytokines that formerly acted only as components of inflammatory defense can venture way out of bounds and become chemical rogues that uncouple bone cell communication.

Osteoimmunology

The ravages of chronic inflammation are currently recognized by doctors as the prime fuel for the catabolic forces of bone loss. Chronic inflammation has on its curriculum vitae a long list of sins that relate to bone loss: disrupter of hormone balance, inhibitor of vitamin D, promoter of the free radicals known as reactive oxygen species (ROS), stimulator of RANKL flow, and igniter of the self-perpetuating match-stick, NF-KB. Today, scientists are examining the physiological interface between our skeletal and immune systems in a new medical field called *osteoimmunology*. From this osteoimmune system of study we've gained a more detailed view of the physiology and biochemistry of bone loss. Some of these important findings are discussed below.

BONE CELLS AND IMMUNE CELLS FORM INSIDE THE BONE MARROW

Bone's macroarchitecture, with its hard outer cortex and hollowed out inside, makes it function like a melding crucible for cells. The marrow inside bone is the birthplace of all your immune cells, as well as all of your bone cells. Bone marrow provides cells the ultimate microenvironment in which to develop and interact. This intimate environment gives the immune system the perfect opportunity to influence bone cells during their process of remodeling. Through the study of stem cells, we now understand how this cellular intimacy, when immersed in chronic inflammation, leads to bone loss.

ADULT STEM CELLS

Stem cells are your body's most basic and unspecialized yet most diversely capable cells. They are the foundation for all the other cells in your body. When tissue cells die, stem cells replace them with new cells. Not only do stem cells have the ability to *differentiate* (a developmental process) along a pathway of increasing specialization, they also retain the ability to make identical copies of themselves, almost indefinitely. These two unique traits provide stem cells with an almost endless capacity to repair your body.

There are three types of stem cells known to populate bone marrow. Two of these are of great concern to us in our study of osteoporosis. *Hematopoietic stem cells* are the first. These can develop into red blood cells, white blood cells, or osteoclasts. The *mesenchymal stem cells* are the second type. These differentiate into either fat cells or osteoblasts. You should try to remember which cells are derived from which type of stem cell. This is because cells derived from a common ancestry respond to similar cytokine signaling, and their differentiation can be dramatically affected by chronic inflammation. This will become important to you as you begin planning nutritional interventions to correct your designated therapeutic targets.

Hematopoietic stem cells. The term "hematopoiesis" means "to make blood," and this is exactly what these stem cells do. When your doctor orders a complete blood count (CBC), he or she is interested in analyzing the blood cells that are of hematopoietic origin—the red blood cells (RBCs) and white blood cells (WBCs). It was only recently discovered that osteoclasts are also formed from this same type of stem cell. Interestingly, the formation of osteoclasts proceeds along the same differentiation pathway as the macrophages and dendritic cells (see figure 4-4). You will soon see why this is so important.

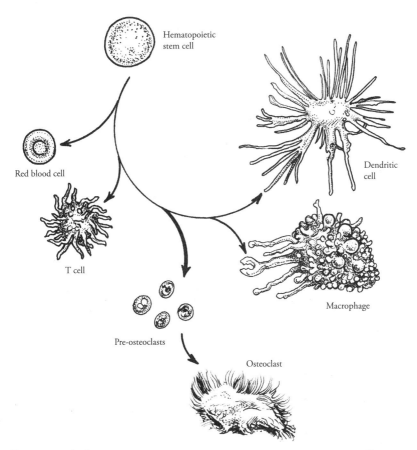

FIGURE 4-4: Differentiation pathways of a hematopoietic stem cell.

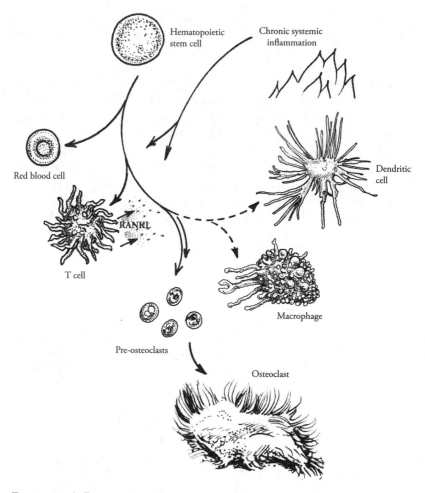

FIGURE 4-5: Chronic inflammation diverts the cell differentiation process away from WBCs and toward osteoclast formation.

Look closely at the differentiation of the hematopoietic stem cell in figure 4-4. There is a fork in the pathway that leads to macrophages and dendritic cells. Taking the third fork to the right leads you to the development of osteoclasts. Now look at figure 4-5 and see what happens when there's chronic inflammation. When the immune system is off balance, the T cells become hyperactive and pump out so much RANKL that a physiological switch is thrown—in error. This switch mechanism diverts the differentiation process of these cells, similar to the way that a switch operator throws a rail switch in a train yard to divert a train from one track to another. The presence of too much RANKL throws a switch that diverts cell differentiation away from the WBCs and toward the development of bone-devouring osteoclasts.

Your job is to do everything you can to prevent this diversion from happening. One clue: Calcium supplementation won't do it. Okay, a second clue: Having a healthy gut, devoid of inflammation and abnormal bacterial overgrowth, is one of the most important steps you can take to reduce systemic inflammation and regain healthy bone.

Mesenchymal stem cells. The second type of stem cells found in your bone marrow are the *mesenchymal stem cells*. These cells are capable of differentiating into either fat cells or osteoblasts (see figure 4-6). Although many people with osteoporosis are underweight and would do well to put on a few pounds, when the pelvic bone of an osteoporotic person is biopsied, it is often filled with too many fat cells and not enough osteoblasts. It is thought that this preponderance of fat cells may be the result of another switch type of mechanism, one that is also manipulated by chronic systemic inflammation.

Dr. Farhad Parhami, from the Cardiology Division of the School of Medicine at the University of California, Los Angeles, showed that diets high in fat contribute not only to heart disease but also to osteoporosis (2003). His research demonstrated that high oxidative stress and the subsequent oxidization of blood lipids (fats) caused mice to lose bone. When these fats were oxidized, they stimulated the production of a regulatory protein called *PPAR-gamma* within the nuclei of stem cells. This protein then caused the differentiation of the mesenchymal stem cells to be diverted away from osteoblast formation and toward fat cell formation (see figure 4-7).

In other words, PPAR-gamma may be the switch operator that throws this second switch and is responsible for the fat accumulation found in the marrow of osteoporotic bone. Not only does this switch reduce the number of osteoblasts, the excess fat crowds out the red blood cells and produces pro-inflammatory cytokines, which bring in even more osteoclasts (Rosen and Bouxsein 2006). When you combine this observation with the suggestion by geriatric expert Dr. William Ershler, of the National Institute on Aging, that cytokine IL-6 can inhibit red blood cell production (2003), it's no wonder that many of my patients with chronic inflammation not only have osteoporosis, they also have anemia.

Bisphosphonates Do Not Stop Chronic Inflammation

Bisphosphonate medications have their place in the treatment of osteoporosis, but they don't reduce inflammation and they don't stop switch operators from throwing switches. Bisphosphonates simply disable osteoclasts and prevent them from resorbing bone. If you've sustained one or more fragility fractures or you are elderly and your BMD is dangerously low, bisphosphonates can help you to reduce your fracture risk. However, these medications carry a side effect that no one ever talks about. When they are taken alone—without the addition of nutritional therapy—the resulting stomach pain, esophagitis, bone and joint pain, and even the fear of osteonecrosis of the jaw all pale in comparison to the lost chance to reduce chronic inflammation.

Using bisphosphonates is like your hiking guide sprinkling fire retardant on a campfire and then leaving the embers smoldering beneath the retardant. Bisphosphonates don't stop the actual mechanisms responsible for the destruction of bone. They don't limit RANKL, NFkB, or PPAR-gamma. They simply harden bones. The insidious forces of inflammation continue smoldering unnoticed and untouched. And just as it takes only a small breeze for embers to spark a fire in nearby tinder, it doesn't take much for chronic inflammation, left untouched, to burst into conflagration and cause chronic degenerative diseases.

LINKING CHRONIC INFLAMMATION AND OXIDATIVE STRESS

Oxidative stress is part of the inflammatory process and vice versa. In their contributions to bone loss, they are inextricably linked. As chronic inflammation becomes more embedded within tissues, it induces more and more oxidative stress, which then creates more inflammation. The more oxidative stress, the more free radicals are produced. The more free radicals, the more tissue damage, and the greater the inflammatory response (see figure 4-8). It's a self-perpetuating process that leads to a progressive accumulation of tissue damage and bone loss.

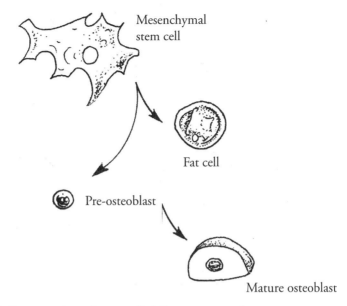

FIGURE 4-6: Mesenchymal stem cell differentiation pathways.

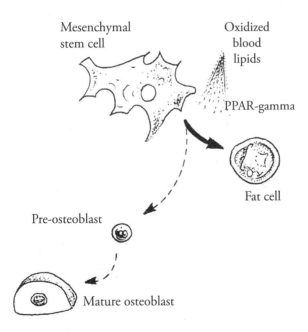

FIGURE 4-7: PPAR-gamma diverts cell differentiation away from osteoblasts and toward fat cells.

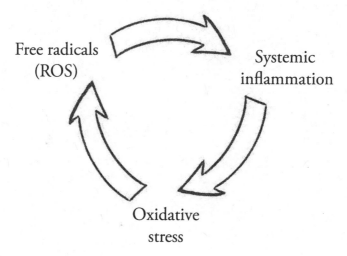

FIGURE 4-8: The inflammatory cycle.

Sources of Inflammation and Oxidative Stress

Poor lifestyle decisions (such as smoking and excessive alcohol consumption), gastrointestinal distress, unhealthy diet choices, hormonal imbalances, toxicity, and stress can all lead to inflammation, oxidative stress, and bone loss. Your number one priority is to reduce as many sources of inflammation and oxidative stress as possible.

GASTROINTESTINAL DISTRESS

The gastrointestinal tract is lined with an estimated 60 to 70 percent of the body's immune defenses. This makes sense when we consider everything that we put into our mouths. Constant activation of the gut's immune defenses is a trigger for chronic inflammation to the rest of the body. Persistent, unexplained abdominal pain, bloating, belching, constipation, diarrhea, gas, foul-smelling stools—these aren't just signs and symptoms of gastrointestinal distress, they are flaming red flags signaling that your gut is fueling your whole body with conflagration.

POOR DIET

A pro-inflammatory diet is one constantly high in sugar, red meat, and processed foods and low in fruits, vegetables, and omega-3 fatty acids. Fruits and vegetables are packed full of antioxidants; if you don't eat them daily, oxidative stress cannot be controlled.

HORMONAL IMBALANCES

Inadequate amounts of sex hormones (estrogen and testosterone), excessive adrenal cortisol, elevated thyroid hormone, high gut-derived serotonin, and the constant overproduction of parathyroid hormone are the major hormonal imbalances that lead to bone loss. They all can be caused by chronic inflammation.

Remember in chapter 3 you learned that the loss of estrogen at menopause leads to the accumulation of ROS free radicals in the bone marrow? Now we know why this causes bone loss. Researchers from Emory University in Atlanta, Georgia, and the University of Udine, in Udine, Italy, recently discovered that marrow high in ROS increases dendritic cell activity fivefold (Grassi et al. 2007). It also activates the T cells. The T cells then release RANKL, which throws the switch diverting the differentiation process away from dendritic cells and toward osteoclasts (look back at figure 4-5). That means that instead of a fivefold increase in dendritic cells, we now have a fivefold increase in osteoclasts. Couple the increase in ROS due to menopause with the high levels of ROS caused by chronic inflammation and oxidative stress, and you can see how osteoclast cell formation (and subsequent bone resorption) would substantially increase and become a direct route to osteoporosis.

TOXICITY, STRESS, AGING, AND INFLAMMATION

Toxins, from both internal and external sources, increase inflammation, free radicals, and oxidative stress. Constant emotional or physical stress and persistent feelings of depression, hostility, or anger are all sources of pro-inflammatory cytokines and contribute to chronic inflammation. Moreover, as we age, our bodies become more inflamed. We get stiffer, have more aches, pains, and memory lapses, and lack the energy we once had. Of course, these are due to the natural deterioration in biological functions; however, they are also the consequences of chronic inflammation.

Biomarkers of Inflammation

Direct laboratory testing of the pro-inflammatory cytokines IL-1, IL-6, and TNF to determine your level of inflammation is possible, but expensive. Tests for the following four biomarkers are much more affordable and are readily available through your doctor.

HOMOCYSTEINE

Typically linked to heart disease, this inflammation biomarker can also be used as an indicator for increased fracture risk. Elevated levels of homocysteine in the blood interfere with the normal cross-linking of bone collagen fibers, which makes them fragile and the skeleton more susceptible to fracture. Blood levels above 8 μmol/L are indicative of inflammation, and when they rise above 15 μmol/L, there is a 2.5-fold increase in fracture risk (Gjesdal et al. 2007).

C-REACTIVE PROTEIN (HIGH SENSITIVITY)

Elevated high sensitivity C-reactive protein (hs-CRP) is positively cor-related to excess production of interleukin-6 (IL-6), chronic inflamma-tion, heart disease, and increased fracture risk (Ganesan et al. 2005). In fact, one study (Ding el al. 2008) showed that abnormally elevated levels of this biomarker predict excess bone resorption and lower BMD. Your blood level of hs-CRP should not be higher than 1.3 mg/L and is best kept below 1.0 mg/L for general health. Another study (Pasco et al. 2006) found a 23 percent increase in fracture risk with each standard deviation increase in hs-CRP, and this was completely independent of bone density. In yet another study (Cauley et al. 2007), when hs-CRP was greater than 3.14 mg/L, a 37 percent increase in fracture risk was seen.

AA TO EPA RATIO

Arachadonic acid (AA) and *eicosapentaenoic acid* (EPA) are essential fatty acids. AA is an omega-6 fatty acid that is considered inflammatory because it fuels the production of pro-inflammatory compounds. High levels are found in red meat and corn products, so you should consume these foods in moderation. EPA is an omega-3 fatty acid that produces anti-inflammatory compounds and is found in high amounts in fatty fish. A typical American diet is far too high in AA and too low in EPA. The ideal ratio of AA to EPA is 1.5 to 1.0, but diets with a ratio of 10 to 1, or even greater, are common. When AA is the predominant fatty acid in the diet, it leads to inflammation. The *AA to EPA ratio* is a blood test that will tell you if you need to reduce dietary AA or increase EPA (or other omega-3s) in your effort to reduce systemic inflammation.

FIBRINOGEN

Fibrinogen is a protein that helps in the formation of blood clots when you've been injured. But when there is chronic systemic inflammation, the body produces excess fibrinogen, which leads to cardiovascular disease. Unlike hs-CRP, which has been directly linked to osteoporosis, fibrinogen can be used only as a general marker of inflammation.

Biomarkers of Oxidative Stress

There are two excellent biomarkers for oxidative stress. The first, *serum lipid peroxides*, can be measured by any laboratory. The second, a marker with the intimidating name of *urine 8-hydroxy-2'-deoxyguanosine* (8OH2dG), is usually tested only at specialty labs (see Resources).

SERUM LIPID PEROXIDES

The fat within your cell membranes is very vulnerable to damage from free radicals. High oxidative stress and the resulting increase in ROS production oxidize fat and release it in the form of lipid peroxides into the blood. The level of lipid peroxides can then be measured as an index of oxidative stress. If you have elevated lipid peroxides, that indicates the fatty membranes surrounding your cells are being damaged. This impairs cell functioning and leads to premature aging. It may also mean that you're producing high amounts of PPAR-gamma, the switch operator that throws the switch to limit osteoblast formation and thus limits the production of bone. This is one reason why oxidative stress is seen as a major contributor to osteoporosis.

URINE 8-HYDROXY-2'-DEOXYGUANOSINE

Don't allow this complicated-sounding compound 8-hydroxy-2'-deoxyguanosine to faze you. And don't let the fact that your doctor probably hasn't ever heard of it sway you from using it to assess your level of oxidative stress. Say it aloud a few times: 8 OH 2 d G, 8 OH 2 d G. This will help you to familiarize yourself with this great test.

When 8OH2dG is elevated in the urine, that indicates not only a heightened level of oxidative stress but actual damage to the genetic material within your cells. How awesome is that? Well, not if it's happening in *your* body. But if you know about it, at least you can do something to reduce it. To have this technology available at your fingertips is like coming to a trailhead and seeing a sign warning of an evil troll up ahead. How fortunate that a kind trail guide thought to post such a sign.

When 8OH2dG is used in combination with testing for lipid peroxides, the two tests will give you a good overall view of your level of oxidative stress. These biomarkers aren't always elevated in osteoporosis (thank goodness), but when they are, and when they can be reduced by proper nutrition, your bone resorption marker, if abnormally elevated, will inevitably fall. This can be very helpful in reducing your fracture risk.

HEART DISEASE AND OSTEOPOROSIS

The link between heart disease and osteoporosis is now well established. One observational study (Tanko et al. 2005) determined that people with osteoporosis had a fourfold increase in their risk for cardiovascular disease. The common thread is chronic inflammation. In addition, atherosclerosis is thought to contribute to bone loss in the hip; it is seen as a type of "bone vascular disease" (Jordan 2005). Chronic inflammation and the atherosclerotic narrowing of small blood vessels prevent oxygen and nutrients from reaching the hip bone. The result—loss of bone density and increased fracture risk (Bagger et al. 2007).

The link between osteoporosis and vascular disease is so strong that it may be prudent to consider low BMD a risk marker for cardiovascular disease. That's a strong statement—but true. Low bone density should be used as a marker for heart disease just as we currently use cholesterol. Be on the safe side. If you have bone loss, ask your doctor to assess your cardiovascular risk.

PUTTING IT ALL TOGETHER—HOW TO REDUCE YOUR INFLAMMATION

You will want to eliminate whatever is causing inflammation and oxidative stress in your life. This means food allergens, microbial overgrowth in your gut, hormonal imbalances, environmental toxins, and emotional stress must all be addressed. They all upset the balance of your immune system's two-armed response and can lead to chronic inflammation and bone loss. Your goal is to do everything you can to reduce excessive RANKL, NF-kB, and PPAR-gamma. Try to follow these recommendations.

Reduce stress. To reduce chronic inflammation, you can start off by reducing stress.

Eat frequently. By not going hungry and eating frequently throughout the day, you will stimulate the growth of healthy bone.

Eliminate food allergens and sensitivities. Your diet can make a huge difference in relieving the inflammation and oxidative stress that lead to bone loss. If you are allergic to any foods, such as wheat, dairy, corn, soy, or eggs, or if you are sensitive to any foods, such as gluten, eliminate them from your diet.

Reduce pro-inflammatory foods. Foods known to increase inflammation should be avoided. These include excessive amounts of red meat, especially from corn-fed cattle raised in feedlots (buy range-fed beef instead), dairy products, refined sugars, saturated fats, hydrogenated and partially hydrogenated fats, and cooking oils made from corn, sunflower, or safflower.

Increase anti-inflammatory foods. Foods with an anti-inflammatory effect and those high in antioxidants, such as green vegetables, fish (rich in omega-3s), berries, seeds, avocados, olive oil, and nuts should be increased. Omega-3 polyunsaturated fatty acids, found in oily fish, hemp seed, canola oil, and flaxseed, help reduce inflammation, moderate the activity of PPAR-gamma, and improve bone health.

Supplement your diet with antioxidants. In addition to dietary changes, there are many natural supplements that can be used to reduce inflammation and oxidative stress. Many have even been shown to reduce bone loss. Osteoporotic women often have low levels of antioxidants, which will increase ROS and activate osteoclastic activity (Maggio et al. 2003). One study (Lean et al. 2003) showed that increasing *glutathione*, the major antioxidant in the body, can prevent bone loss in estrogen-deficient rodents. This is an amazing finding considering how important estrogen is for maintaining bone.

In this study, the glutathione was able to reduce ROS and the pro-inflammatory cytokine TNF so dramatically that, even with low estrogen, bone resorption was curtailed. Another study (Prouillet et al. 2004) demonstrated that antioxidants increased bone formation by reducing the catabolic effects of chronic low-level inflammation and oxidative stress. If you are postmenopausal, what this means is that supplementing your diet with antioxidants may help reduce inflammation and preserve your skeleton, despite your low levels of estrogen.

The following nutrients are capable of antioxidant activity and increasing glutathione in the body: vitamins C, E, and K, zinc, selenium, manganese, molybdenum, DHEA, ubiquinone (coenzyme Q10), alpha-lipoic acid, N-acetyl cysteine, milk thistle, carotenoids, quercetin, rutin, ginger, resveratrol, leucine, taurine, lycopene, and curcumin. These are all capable of reducing oxidative stress and NF-KB, and therefore inflammation.

- Curcumin not only reduces inflammation and oxidative stress (Balasubramanyam et al. 2003), it also inhibits lipid peroxidation and reduces NF-KB (Bengmark 2006), which is important for inhibiting RANKL, and therefore bone resorption. This makes curcumin a good choice if your bone resorption marker is elevated, or your osteocalcin is depressed, especially if your joints are feeling cranky from chronic inflammation.

- Lycopene not only has been shown to reduce oxidative stress, but in a study with postmenopausal women (Rao et al. 2207), it also reduced bone resorption markers.

- The omega-3 fatty acids DHA and EPA reduce pro-inflammatory cytokines and help reduce bone loss.

- I've found that alpha-lipoic acid, N-acetyl cysteine, and milk thistle make a great combination for reducing abnormally elevated bone resorption markers.

Use probiotics. Supplementation with *Lactobacillus* and *Bifidobacterium* species of probiotics helps to promote gastrointestinal health and reduce systemic inflammation.

Regulate kinase enzymes. When messages from signaling molecules such as pro-inflammatory cytokines or RANKL contact a cell, it's the job of *kinase enzymes* to relay those messages to the cell's interior. There, the cell's nucleus responds to the kinase signals by turning its genetic programming on or off. Just about all of the biological processes within cells are activated or dampened in this way. This includes the lighting or dimming of the inflammatory matchsticks of NF-KB. It also includes the extent to which an osteoclast responds to RANKL, and how powerfully a bone-building osteoblast will respond to vitamin D. All of these cell responses are regulated by kinase enzymes.

This is important because kinase regulation can be modified by certain supplements. For example, there are medicinal herbs called *selective kinase response modulators* (SKRMs) that help dampen inflammation and positively affect bone cells by moderating the signals of kinase enzymes. Recently, SKRMs have been shown to help reduce osteoclastic bone resorption (Tobe et al. 1997) and increase osteoblastic bone formation (Effenberger et al. 2005)

Berberine, traditionally used as an anti-inflammatory and antibacterial herb, is a SKRM, and some spectacular research from Korea indicates that it is good for your skeleton. In a study at the University of Toyama, Japan, Li et al. (2003) showed that berberine can inhibit osteoclastic activity and increase the BMD of osteoporotic mice. Another study (Hu et al. 2008) further defined berberine's actions on bone as having the ability to balance kinase signaling when RANKL levels are too high. This results in less NF-κB production in the osteoclasts, and therefore less bone resorption. But berberine's benefits don't stop there.

Remember the second switch mechanism, illustrated above in figure 4-7? It showed how PPAR-gamma from oxidative stress diverts the differentiation pathway of mesenchymal stem cells away from osteoblasts and toward the formation of fat cells. Berberine represses PPAR-gamma's ability to interfere with this pathway, and therefore limits fat cell production in bone marrow (Huang et al. 2006). A recent study (Lee et al. 2008) showed that berberine actually stimulates osteoblasts to build bone.

Although these studies have been performed only on animals, berberine appears to have promise for treating humans. The fact that it both reduces bone resorption and increases bone formation is astounding. Ongoing research at the Functional Medicine Research Center in Gig Harbor, Washington, has shown that a supplemental combination of vitamins D and K with berberine and another SKRM (rho-iso-alpha acid) was able to reduce bone turnover in postmenopausal women. This was demonstrated by a reduction of urine NTX and a normalization of osteocalcin levels (Joseph Lamb, MD, 2008, personal communication).

Rho-iso-alpha acid (RIAA), an extract made from hops, reduces inflammation (Hall et al. 2008) through NF-κB pathways and has the potential to prevent bone loss and increase bone formation by modulating kinase enzyme activity. In addition to RIAA, there are several flavonoid compounds also found in minute quantities in hops that have demonstrated positive effects on the skeleton. For example, researchers from Oregon State University have isolated a biologically active molecule called *xanthohumol* that has powerful antioxidant activity. It has also been shown to prevent oxidation of LDLs (Stevens et al. 2003) and inhibit bone resorption (Tobe et al. 1997). Stay on the lookout for these compounds and others, such as tetrahydro-iso-alpha acids, and the potent phytoestrogen 8-prenylnaringenin, as future research continues to define their medical benefits.

Recommended Protocol for Reducing Inflammation

I recommend the following supplementation for my patients with elevated biomarkers of inflammation and oxidative stress: vitamin C (500 to 1,000 mg/day); vitamin E (200 to 400 IU/day of mixed tocopherols); vitamin K (K$_1$ and K$_2$ MK-4 and MK-7 450 mcg to 5 mg/day); alpha-lipoic acid (300 to 600 mg/day—not recommended for people with gastroesophageal reflux disease (GERD)); coenzyme Q10 (100 mg/day); milk thistle (400 mg/day); N-acetyl cysteine (500 to 1,000 mg, three times a day); taurine (1 to 3 g/day); fish oil (2 to 3 g/day); berberine (500 mg/day, or 1,000 mg/day short-term for those with intestinal dysbiosis, a condition of microbial imbalances); rho-iso-alpha acids (500 mg/day); probiotics (3 to 20 billion/day); and DHEA (25 mg/day), when indicated.

Note: As with all antioxidant therapy, excess supplementation should be avoided. Antioxidants can actually turn into pro-oxidants, leading to greater oxidative stress. Moreover, for those of my patients who are taking anticoagulant (blood-thinning) medications, such as warfarin (Coumadin), I am cautious about supplementing with vitamin K. If you're currently taking a blood thinner, be sure to talk to your doctor before supplementing with vitamin K.

Why not use NSAIDS (nonsteroidal anti-inflammatory drugs) to reduce chronic inflammation and improve bone health? You may be wondering why anti-inflammatory medications like ibuprofen can't be used to reduce bone loss related to chronic inflammation. The reason is that these medications are designed to reduce acute, not chronic, inflammation. Therefore, they do nothing to slow down the underlying mechanisms of bone loss.

■ *Ms. Cody*

Let's take a look at Ms. Cody's situation. At the age of forty-eight, she was concerned about osteoporosis and came in for a checkup. I noted several risk factors for osteoporosis on her intake form. As a teenager, Ms. Cody had been both anorexic and bulimic. She had a history of depression and smoked a pack of cigarettes a day, and her mother had suffered a hip fracture from osteoporosis at the age of seventy-two. Ms. Cody's father had died from heart disease at the age of sixty-six, and although this was not technically a risk factor for osteoporosis, I did take note of it. Ms. Cody also checked off several telling signs and symptoms: frequent muscle cramps in her legs, insomnia, joint pains, irritability, and intermittent constipation.

My examination of Ms. Cody revealed the following: She was five feet and six inches tall, weighed 130 pounds, was having regular periods, and had a slightly elevated blood pressure and heart rate. She did not complain of digestive problems, and there was no tenderness or swelling in her abdomen. Her mouth showed the beginnings of periodontal disease. I noted small bumps, like coarse sandpaper, on the backs of her arms, and some dandruff, both indicating a need for essential fatty acids. Ms. Cody also had slight creases in her earlobes, a possible sign of vascular changes that would indicate a risk of cardiovascular disease.

Previous X-rays of Ms. Cody's spine showed no spinal abnormalities, but what caught my eye were the small ash-white specks floating within the soft tissues next to her bones. They were the signs that her tissues were beginning to calcify, a warning flag that her body was not putting calcium into its proper place—her bones. There was even a sprinkling of these specks on her abdominal aorta—an ominous sign for someone her age—signaling that this major artery was beginning to harden. Arterial calcification and atherosclerosis are frequently observed in people with osteoporosis (Hofbauer et al. 2007). Because of Ms. Cody's family history of heart disease and osteoporosis, it was evident that she needed a cardiovascular evaluation and a DXA exam.

Ms. Cody's DXA and Laboratory Evaluation

While waiting for her DXA results, I asked Ms. Cody to bring in her old medical records. Coincidently, she had just had her yearly physical examination and had been tested for cholesterol levels. I wanted to see if these tests revealed anything useful. This is what I found: Ms. Cody's laboratory test results showed that her total cholesterol was high, her LDL cholesterol was high, and her HDL cholesterol was low.

Clearly, Ms. Cody had a less than stellar cholesterol assessment. It was plain to see that she was at high risk for cardiovascular disease. But I was also interested in her cholesterol levels for another reason: for their relationship to her skeletal physiology. Elevated LDLs (the bad cholesterol) have been correlated to increased bone loss, and HDLs (the good cholesterol) are known to be involved in building bone. In Ms.

Cody's case, neither of these cholesterol markers was conducive to good bone health. I was glad that I ordered the DXA, even though Ms. Cody was only forty-eight years old. Unfortunately, Ms. Cody's DXA exam revealed that she had osteoporosis. Her lumbar spine T score was -3.1 and her hips averaged -2.9.

LABORATORY TESTS: THE BASIC CORE

I immediately ordered the basic core of laboratory tests for osteoporosis, which consists of the following tests: comprehensive metabolic panel (CMP), complete blood count (CBC), vitamin D [25(OH)D], urine pH (morning), urine calcium (twenty-four hour sample), celiac profile, and an N-telopeptide (NTX) test.

LABORATORY TESTS: INFLAMMATION AND OXIDATIVE STRESS

Because of Ms. Cody's extensive bone loss and cardiovascular risk, I wanted to evaluate her for inflammation and oxidative stress, so I ordered the following tests: homocysteine; hs-CRP; lipid peroxides; and 8OH2dG. I chose homocysteine and hs-CRP because they are markers of inflammation and they've been directly linked to osteoporosis. Given Ms. Cody's cardiovascular risk, I also thought it important to evaluate her level of oxidative stress by testing her for lipid peroxides and 8OH2dG.

I already knew that her low HDL level might be impacting her ability to form bone, but if the oxidative stress markers were abnormal, her elevated LDL would also become a direct concern to her skeletal health. The reason for this is that the oxidation of LDLs from oxidative stress can lead to bone loss (Parhami et al. 2002). (Remember PPAR-gamma, the switch operator?)

Ms. Cody's Assessment and Treatment

Ms. Cody's teenage struggle with anorexia may have prevented her from reaching optimal peak bone mass, but it did not explain the severity of her current low bone density. We had a lot of information; we just needed to organize it and formulate a treatment plan. Together, Ms. Cody and I sat down and filled out her therapeutic targets form.

MS. CODY'S OSTEOPOROTIC INDICATIONS AND THERAPEUTIC TARGETS

- *Osteoporosis*: Spine: -3.1; hips: -2.9; DXA date 3/14/2005. *Therapeutic plan*: A basic bone-support product to provide calcium (microcrystalline hydroxyapatite complex); magnesium; vitamins C, D, B12, K, and folic acid; boron; trace amounts of strontium; zinc; manganese; copper; and silicon. Basic nutritional support from a multivitamin-mineral complex (with vitamin A from mixed carotenoids, not retinol); whey protein powder (20 g/day); and fish oil or krill oil.

Her risk factors were as follows:

- Anorexic and bulimic as a teenager, indicating a possible failure to reach peak bone mass.

- Maternal history of osteoporosis with hip fracture, indicating a possible genetic predisposition for osteoporosis.

- Cigarette smoking. *Plan*: Reduce use or quit.

- Mild periodontal disease, which is often correlated to bone loss.

- Sedentary lifestyle. *Plan*: Begin exercise program.

- Depression. *Plan*: General nutritional support, B complex, and S-adenosinemethionine (SAMe).

MS. CODY'S SIGNS AND SYMPTOMS AND TREATMENT PLANS

- *Dandruff*: Essential fatty acids.

- *Bumps on backs of arms*: Essential fatty acids.

- *Leg cramps*: Magnesium (600 mg/day).

- *Intermittent constipation*: Magnesium.

- *Soft-tissue calcifications noted on X-rays*: Vitamin K (3 mg/day).

- *Rapid pulse*: Essential fatty acids, amino acids, and magnesium.

- *Multiple joint pains*: Curcumin.

- *Irritability*: Magnesium.

- *Fatigue*: Overall nutritional support.

MS. CODY'S CORE LAB TESTS, RESULTS, INDICATIONS, AND THERAPEUTIC PLANS

- *Test*: Comprehensive metabolic panel, 4/4/2005.
  Results: Cholesterol: high; Calcium: low-normal. Plan: Reduce oxidative stress, supplement with magnesium.

- *Test*: CBC, 4/4/2005.
  Results: Normal.

- *Test*: Vitamin D, 4/4/2005.
  Results: 36 ng/ml, normal.

- *Test*: Urine pH, 4/4 thru 4/10/2005.
  Results: Low (an average of 5.6). Plan: Increase fruits and vegetables, reduce red meat consumption, and supplement with potassium bicarbonate (600 mg/day).

- *Test*: Urine calcium (24-hour), 4/4/2005.
  Results: High (324 mg). Plan: Increase fruits and vegetables, reduce salt intake, and supplement with boron, potassium bicarbonate, and vitamin K.

- *Test*: Celiac profile, 4/4/2005.
  Results: Normal.

- *Test*: N-telopeptide, 4/4/2005.
  Results: High (138 nmolBCE/mmol). Indication: Rapid bone loss.

MS. CODY'S INFLAMMATION BIOMARKERS, RESULTS, AND THERAPEUTIC PLANS

- *Test*: Homocysteine, 4/4/2005.
  Results: High (16 µmol/L). Plan: Supplement with vitamins B2, B6, and B12 and folate.

- *Test*: Hs-CRP, 4/4/2005.
  Results: High (1.7 mg/L). Plan: Reduce inflammation by supplementing with fish oil (3 g/day) or krill oil, vitamin C (1 g/day), alpha-lipoic acid (300 mg/day) with biotin, N-acetyl cysteine, taurine, milk thistle, and curcumin.

MS. CODY'S OXIDATIVE STRESS BIOMARKERS, RESULTS, AND THERAPEUTIC PLANS

- *Test*: Lipid peroxides 4/4/2005.
  Results: High. Plan: Eat more fruits and vegetables and supplement with vitamin C, vitamin E (high gamma, mixed tocopherols), alpha-lipoic acid, and N-acetyl cysteine.

- *Test*: 8OH2dG, 4/4/2005.
  Results: High. Plan: Same as for lipid peroxides.

MS. CODY'S OTHER LAB TESTS, RESULTS, AND THERAPEUTIC PLANS

- *Test*: IGF-1, 4/4/2005.
  Results: Low. Plan: Improve sleep, start moderate exercise program, and supplement with whey protein and zinc (20 mg/day).

- *Test*: LDL cholesterol, 2/3/2005.
  Results: High. Plan: Reduce oxidative stress, exercise, stop smoking, decrease consumption of trans and saturated fats and increase monounsaturated fats and fish oil.

- *Test*: HDL cholesterol, 2/3/2005.
  Results: Low. Plan: Same as for LDL cholesterol.

The markers for Ms. Cody's bone loss pointed directly to low-level metabolic acidosis and chronic systemic inflammation. Her inflammatory and oxidative stress biomarkers were elevated, indicating that excessive ROS were fueling osteoclasts and toasting her bones. No wonder her NTX was so high.

I began Ms. Cody's treatment with a general bone-specific support supplement (which included calcium, magnesium and other minerals), a multivitamin-mineral complex, whey protein, and fish and krill oil.

Curcumin and antioxidants were added to help lower her inflammation and oxidative stress. Diet changes (vegetables and more vegetables) along with boron, potassium, and vitamin K supplementation would reduce the calcium loss seen in her urine. The 1,200 mg per day of calcium and 600 mg per day of magnesium would not only help her skeleton, it would also reduce her muscle cramping, constipation, and irritability.

It's not just your muscles and bones that require protein; it's also necessary for hormone production. To ensure that Ms. Cody's estrogen production was optimal, I recommended that she consume whey protein in addition to the quality protein in her diet. Since whey is a high-quality protein that has been shown to increase BMD, I recommended that she consume a shake made from fruit, yogurt, and 20 mg whey protein powder once a day between two meals. Note: Whey protein increases insulin secretion. Therefore, if you have a glucose-control problem, such as diabetes, a better protein choice might be rice, soy, pea, or hemp.

Over the following year, Ms. Cody's NTX steadily declined. Indeed, all her therapeutic targets showed improvement on repeat testing. Ms. Cody was feeling so much better that she even had the energy to attack her addiction to cigarettes. With her reduced fracture risk and improved cardiovascular health, Ms. Cody told me she felt twenty years younger.

EXERCISE 4.1: WHAT ARE YOUR THERAPEUTIC TARGETS?

Divide the first page of your journal into three columns. Each column will take a separate heading. The heads are Bone Status, DXA Date, and Therapeutic Plan. Even though you and your doctor may prefer to add or eliminate certain supplements, you can copy the following information as a good starting point under the column head for Therapeutic Plan: a basic bone-support product that provides—calcium (microcrystalline hydroxyapatite complex); magnesium; vitamins C, D, B$_{12}$, K, and folic acid; boron; strontium; zinc; manganese; copper; and silicon. Add basic nutritional support in the form of a multivitamin complex (with vitamin A source from mixed carotenoids, not retinol); whey protein powder (20 g/day); and fish oil or krill oil.

Then, on the next two pages, copy the following headings. Use two columns on each page, and over time, fill in the relevant information on the blank pages under the appropriate headings. On the first page (sample page 2), write Osteoporosis Risk Factors and Indication/Therapeutic Plan; and on the second page (sample page 3), write Signs and Symptoms and Therapeutic Plan.

When you have completed those two pages, take the next four pages to write in the following heads, but this time divide the pages into three columns instead of two. The headings for the first page (sample page 4) will be Core Lab Tests (and Dates), Results, and Indication/Therapeutic Plan. Under Core Lab Tests and Dates, pencil in the following core lab tests: comprehensive metabolic panel (CMP), date; complete blood count (CBC), date; vitamin D [25(OH)D], date; urine pH (morning), date; urine calcium (24-hour sample), date; celiac profile, date; and resorption biomarker, date. It is important that you copy the core lab tests to this blank page because that will help to ensure you will get the necessary core lab tests.

Finally, take three more blank pages in your journal and copy the following three sets of heads at the top of each page (sample pages 5, 6, and 7). You can fill them in as you progress in your treatment.

1. Inflammation Biomarkers, Date; Results; and Therapeutic Plan

2. Oxidative Stress Biomarkers, Date; Results; and Therapeutic Plan.

3. Other Lab Tests, Date; Results; and Therapeutic Plan

SAMPLE JOURNAL PAGES FOR EXERCISE 4.1

Bone Status	DXA Date	Therapeutic Plan

Page 1

Osteoporosis Risk Factors	Indication/Therapeutic Plan

Page 2

Signs and Symptoms	Therapeutic Plan

Page 3

Core Lab Tests Dates	Results	Indication/ Therapeutic Plan
Comprehensive Metabolic Panel (CMP), Date		
Complete Blood Count, Date		
Vitamin D [25(OH)D], Date		
Urine pH (morning), Date		
Urine calcium (24-hour sample), Date		
Celiac profile, Date		
Resorption biomarker, Date		

Page 4

Inflammation Biomarkers	Date	Results	Therapeutic Plan

Page 5

Oxidative Stress Biomarkers	Date	Results	Therapeutic Plan

Page 6

Other Lab Tests	Date	Results	Therapeutic Plan

Page 7

THE PLACE TO START

In case you're starting to think that osteoporosis is very complicated, you are right; it is. Trying to pinpoint exactly what is causing your bone loss can sometimes be overwhelming. In fact, you may never fully understand all of the reasons for your osteoporosis. But at least you are now well aware of the hazards of burning embers. Just hang in there. You are much better equipped now that you understand how to skirt forest fires and avoid setting them. Fill out the therapeutic targets form and, one by one, try to improve things. You will wind up with better health and reduced fracture risk.

CHAPTER FIVE

Your Digestive System: Gateway to Health or Quagmire for Bone Loss?

You had to run hard there for a while to escape the forest fire set by careless hikers. Now you're a little lost but at least you're safe—for the time being. You find yourself in a very dense section of the forest. In front of you lies an overgrown gateway leading to a dark, tunnel-like trail that forks immediately. What you don't know is that one path leads to an open clearing, radiant with energy, with a source of water so pure that it's almost like the fountain of youth. The other path, unfortunately, is bordered by bushes with sharp, nasty thorns, and is frequented by horrible goblins. It eventually empties into an impassable, marshy quagmire so toxic that it will suck the very life out of an unsuspecting hiker. Your digestive system can take on the appearance of either of these two paths. It's up to you to choose the one that leads to skeletal health and to bypass the path that can lead to chronic systemic inflammation and disease.

THE ANATOMY OF DIGESTION

Your digestive system consists of the *gastrointestinal (GI) tract* and the organs that have evolved specifically for the digestion of food. The GI tract begins at your mouth, travels twenty to twenty-five tortuous feet as a convoluted muscular tube, and ends at the anus. Your digestive organs are your teeth, tongue, salivary glands, stomach, gallbladder, liver, and pancreas. These specialized organs and tissues help to break down food into smaller particles for better absorption through the GI tract wall.

Your Gastrointestinal Tract

The wall of your GI tract is a specialized tissue formed by just a single layer of cells. This tissue, called *mucosa,* is all that separates your insides from the outside world. Amazingly, your mucosa is able to be absorptive, like a sponge soaking up nutrients, while at the same time maintaining a protective barrier against pathogens and alien molecules. Absorbent yet impenetrable—a task that is possible only when your mucosa is healthy. The GI tract's mucosal cells have tiny, fingerlike projections called *villi.* When these delicate structures are looked at under a microscope, they give the inside of your intestines the look and texture of velvety willow catkins. It is through these villi that your intestines are provided with a huge surface area from which to absorb nutrients.

In addition to being absorbed through villi, molecules enter your body through the connections or *tight junctions* that hold mucosal cells firmly against each other. Once thought to be unyielding, impenetrable bonds between cells, these tight junctions—gatekeepers, if you will—are now known to be dynamic, complex structures that open and close depending on the stimulus.

Certain nutrients, nerve signals, and inflammatory molecules trigger the release of a protein called *zonulin* from the mucosal cells. Zonulin stimulates the tight junctions to temporarily open, thus allowing the entry of molecules into your body (Arrieta, Bistritz, and Meddings 2006). In a healthy body, this dual mucosal system of absorptive villi and dynamic tight junctions is a perfect system that allows nutrients to enter but remains a barrier to pathogens.

If for any reason this GI cell barrier is breached by undesirable molecules or pathogens, the mucosa can mount an immediate immunological defense. Within the mucosa are clusters of lymph tissue that serve as immunological checkpoints. From these clusters, sentry white blood cells (WBCs) scrutinize everything that passes through your intestines, and if they sense a threat, macrophages and dendritic cells attack and mount an immediate, inflammatory response.

Your Organs of Digestion

The miracle of digestion, where foods are converted into energy and the building blocks for our tissues, begins with chewing and ends with elimination. When food is swallowed into the stomach, hydrochloric acid (HCl) breaks it down further and finishes the job of killing potential pathogens. The HCl then activates the release of digestive enzymes for the food's further breakdown. Together, the HCl and digestive enzymes turn proteins into peptides and amino acids, complex carbohydrates into simple sugars, and fats into free fatty acids. This all happens so that just about anything you consume can miraculously be transformed into you.

IMPAIRED DIGESTION

Gulping down your food and eating a low-fiber diet are terrible for your digestion. Just chewing your food longer will aid your mucosal cells in their ability to absorb vital nutrients. And eating lots of fiber helps to transport food down through your GI tract. Without fiber, the rhythmic intestinal contractions of *peristalsis* have a tough time squeezing food through the long pipeline of the GI tract, so it just sits there and rots.

The stomach's secretion of HCl is also a key element of the digestive process. As we age, HCl production decreases and our digestion suffers. By the time we reach our seventies, stomach acid secretion may be only a fraction of what it was when we were forty. Medications such as proton-pump inhibitors (PPIs) reduce HCl secretion. Reduced stomach acid, whether due to aging or medications, compromises digestion, reduces nutrient absorption, and contributes to bone loss.

Signs and Symptoms of Impaired Digestion

Poor digestion and the putrefaction of food in the intestines provide both a smorgasbord and a breeding ground for pathogens. As bacteria chow down, they also release an embarrassing amount of gas. The gas builds up in the intestines, causing pain, belching, bloating, and flatulence. These unpleasant reactions are informing you that your digestion is impaired, that your gut is filling up with toxins, and that your ability to absorb nutrients is being compromised. I'm always amazed when I see a patient who brings in lumbar or abdominal X-rays ordered by another doctor, and the films are riddled with the silhouettes of copious intestinal gas. My amazement is not that the patient has gas—many people have unhealthy digestive systems—but I am taken aback by the fact that no one has informed the patient of this obvious sign of ill health.

If you're experiencing symptoms of digestive distress immediately after eating, it's usually a sign that you need HCl. The remedy is simple: supplement each meal with HCl tablets. This will aid your digestive process and stimulate the release of all the other necessary digestive enzymes. If your symptoms are more delayed, say, two to four hours after a meal, try some digestive enzymes and also be on the lookout for food allergies. When there is an imbalance in the number or species of gut microflora, it is referred to as *dysbiosis*. This condition can result from too many "bad" microorganisms or too few of the "good" ones. Either case can be a prime source of inflammation.

GUT MICROFLORA

More than five hundred species of microorganisms live in your GI tract. Some form colonies and are important to your survival, others just pass through on a joyride, and still others lie in wait for the opportunity to colonize. The "good" bacteria, such as various types, or strains, of *Lactobacillus* and *Bifidobacterium*, are so important that together they are considered an essential organ of your body. These are referred to as your *commensal microbes,* and when you are healthy, they colonize your gut in high numbers. Commensal microbes aid in the digestion of food, elimination of toxins, manufacture of nutrients such as vitamin K_2, and prevention of overcolonization by opportunistic organisms or dangerous pathogens.

Low HCl production and poor digestion, PPI medications, and the use of antibiotics all increase your chances that opportunistic and pathogenic bacteria, fungi (yeast), or parasites will set up a squatters' camp in your GI tract. These microbes are the same goblins that haunt the trail to the marshy quagmire.

DYSBIOSIS AND THE ACTIVATION OF THE IMMUNE SYSTEM

Pathogens not destroyed by stomach acid are met in the small intestine by a second line of defense. A virtual army of immune cells capable of destroying any microbial threat is waiting for them. To put it bluntly, the intestines can be filthy quarters, and your immunity needs to be operating on all cylinders to keep you healthy.

Toll-like receptors. Macrophages, dendritic cells, and some of your gut's mucosal cells are equipped with microbe identification scanners called *toll-like receptors.* These specialized receptors enable the WBCs and mucosal cells to scan the structural patterns on microbes and assess their identity. When a pattern is identified as bad, the microbe is immediately destroyed. Patterns belonging to good bacteria evoke no immune response at all. The more bad patterns recognized, the more heated the skirmishes become. As long as antigens continue to activate the toll-like receptors, the immune system continues to respond.

Pathogens can be sneaky fellows. They've devised intricately covert tactics to gain entry into your body. Some excrete chemicals that stimulate the release of zonulin to open the tight junctions. Like bad guys with the password to a bank vault, some pathogens have learned how to penetrate the GI tract's mucosal barrier. But as they pass through the tight junctions, dendritic cells, macrophages, and a powerful inflammatory response greet them. However, if the breach becomes chronic, the mucosal lining will be damaged and the intestinal wall will begin to leak.

A chronically inflamed digestive tract causes tight junctions to separate permanently, forming gaps through which partially digested food particles and microbes can pass. Now, instead of being a protective barrier, this "leaky gut," properly referred to as *intestinal permeability,* becomes a portal to ill health. The particulate and microbial toxins that filter through these newly opened gaps set off allergic reactions, which are a constant source of inflammation that insidiously permeates the entire body.

Oral tolerance. A healthy gut wall and an intestine full of commensal micro-organisms do not promote an inflammatory response. The toll-like receptors lazily check the identification of the *Lactobacillus* and *Bifidobacterium* species all day and night and, with no sign of danger, the receptors practically fall asleep. In this scenario, the tight junctions remain functional, opening for nutrients yet remaining closed to pathogens. Everything is so calm and tolerant that even minor irritants are able to pass through the digestive tract without setting any fires. This is good.

It's like a soldier knowing when to pull the trigger and when to just accept the jeers and taunts of angry but harmless citizens. Such tolerance by soldiers prevents needless battles. In the gut, this same type of acceptance of minor irritants is called *oral tolerance,* and it helps to prevent unnecessary inflammation. This muted immune response to normal microorganisms and harmless antigens is important for maintaining an intact intestinal wall and the health of the whole body. The key to oral tolerance is maintaining a gut full of good bacteria. Peaceful border control can be encouraged by supplementing your diet with a daily source of probiotics containing strains of *Lactobacillus* and *Bifidobacterium* (see "Reinoculate" near the end of this chapter).

In addition to probiotics, estrogen and vitamin D also help to maintain oral tolerance. For women, it's critical to maintain intestinal health during the menopausal years, when estrogen levels decline sharply. It's not unusual for a woman's oral tolerance to decline during these years. This may be hard to believe, but improving oral tolerance can be done simply by taking a walk in the sun. Vitamin D doesn't just increase your calcium absorption; it also calms your GI tract's immune system.

Breakdown of oral tolerance leads to chronic inflammation. When oral tolerance breaks down, the immune system goes on constant high alert. This creates a continuous outflow of pro-inflammatory cytokines from the intestinal mucosa. In this situation, inflammation from intestinal permeability doesn't stay local to the GI tract; it becomes systemic, increasing the level of pro-inflammatory cytokines in the body and contributing to inflammation-related chronic disease. In the case of osteoporosis, GI tract inflammation can be a potential source of hordes of T cells that release RANKL and throw the switch to encourage osteoclast cell formation.

In 1983, two Australian scientists, Drs. Robin Warren and Barry Marshall, discovered that a stomach infection by the bacteria *Helicobacter pylori* was the cause of peptic and duodenal ulcers. Since then, this bacterium has been implicated in cancer, heart disease, and, yes, even osteoporosis. Its overgrowth is a source of constant inflammation and systemic elevation of levels of the pro-inflammatory cytokines IL-6 and TNF. It should be no surprise that a study (Figura et al. 2005) showed that patients with *H. pylori* infection exhibited increased levels of the bone resorption marker NTX and, hence, had a greater risk for developing osteoporosis.

As I've explained previously, insufficient secretion of stomach acid allows the overcolonization of microorganisms. This is certainly the case with infection by *H. pylori*. Low stomach acid, whether due to genetics, aging, poor nutrition, or PPI medications, will increase your vulnerability to infection by *H. pylori*.

DIAGNOSING DYSBIOSIS

Dysbiosis causes signs and symptoms similar to poor digestion: abdominal pain, belching, bloating, and gas. Fungal overgrowth such as candida yeast can cause additional signs and symptoms: thrush (white-coated tongue), recurring vaginal infections, jock itch, athlete's foot, fingernail infections, or an itchy anus. In addition, dysbiosis should be considered when there are nonspecific changes in laboratory biomarkers. For example, when your doctor looks at the results from your complete blood count (CBC), he or she may find that you are mildly anemic from poor absorption of iron, or have an elevated mean corpuscular volume (MCV), which is indicative of a vitamin B_{12} or folate insufficiency. These may be not just random deficiencies but indications that you're not absorbing nutrients efficiently. Dysbiosis is a frequent contributor to malabsorption.

Specialty labs have an array of tests available for diagnosing dysbiosis. A stool analysis, the hydrogen breath test, the urine organic acids test, and the lactulose-mannitol test can all be useful in determining the extent and cause of microbial imbalance. *H. pylori* can be specifically diagnosed through breath testing, serum antibodies, and stool analysis. If you have osteoporosis and are experiencing digestive problems, talk with your doctor about which test would be most helpful in diagnosing your problem.

GLUTEN SENSITIVITY: A COMMON CAUSE OF BONE LOSS

You have just read about how poor digestion and the overgrowth of microbes can contribute to malabsorption, localized gut inflammation, and systemic inflammation. Food sensitivities and allergic responses to food can cause similar responses. Sensitivity to the gluten protein found in many grains is a leading cause of malabsorption, inflammation, and bone loss.

Celiac Disease

Celiac disease (also referred to as celiac sprue or gluten-sensitive enteropathy) is an autoimmune disease caused by sensitivity to the gluten protein found in wheat, barley, rye and other grains. It's *not* a food allergy. Celiac disease is triggered by a genetically based, immune reaction to gluten initiated by T cells. This intestinal malabsorptive disorder is classically marked by symptoms of diarrhea, gas, bloating, and fatty stools.

When someone is genetically susceptible, the villi of his or her mucosal cells *atrophy*, or shrivel away, in response to gluten-containing grains. This reduces nutrient absorption capability and is the reason why iron-deficient anemia and osteoporosis from calcium and vitamin D deficiency are both commonly seen in people with celiac disease.

Although gluten, in the form of antibody-gluten complexes, can damage mucosal villi and then permeate the gut wall through its cell membranes (Matysiak-Budnik et al. 2008), large quantities of gluten can also enter the body through tight junctions. These structural junctions that firmly hold the intestines' mucosal cells together can open temporarily in response to a regulating protein called zonulin. In certain individuals, gluten can be a powerful stimulator of zonulin release, thereby increasing gut wall permeability. This increased permeability is a problem because it allows the large gluten molecules to enter the body, where they set off an inflammatory immune response.

The diagnosis of celiac disease is easily made when there are obvious signs and symptoms. But many people have "silent" gluten sensitivity with no obvious gastrointestinal involvement. These people often go undiagnosed. The National Institutes of Health has estimated that approximately 1 percent of the U.S. population suffers from celiac disease (James 2005), and one study (Stenson et al. 2005) determined that 3 to 4 percent of people with osteoporosis have celiac disease. That is a huge percentage. Another study (Taranta et al. 2004) estimated that, for at least 30 percent of those with celiac disease, their osteoporosis is severe.

Gluten sensitivity has now been linked to disorders other than those caused by villi atrophication and malabsorption. With our new understanding that gluten has the ability to open tight junctions and cause systemic inflammation, regardless of its effects on mucosal villi, we are realizing that more people are being adversely affected by gluten than the statistics show. Some cases of diabetes, inflammation of the thyroid gland, Sjögren's syndrome, and even neurological and psychiatric disorders also appear to be linked to gluten (Helms 2005). So common is gluten sensitivity in osteoporotic patients that laboratory screening is now recommended for anyone with bone loss, whether or not the person has gastrointestinal signs or symptoms (Stenson et al. 2005).

EXERCISE 5.1: Become Aware of Gluten Sensitivity

Gluten sensitivity can present in an almost endless array of signs and symptoms. I've listed some of the most common ones below. Highlight or circle any that you may be experiencing. If you have osteoporosis, you should not rely on the presence of symptoms to indicate the need for testing. Ask your doctor to test you for gluten sensitivity if that hasn't already been done.

The following lists some of the signs and symptoms of gluten sensitivity: diarrhea or loose stools, abdominal pain, bloating or abdominal distention, excessive gas, pale and foul-smelling stool, irritability, depression, weight loss, anemia, fatigue, general weakness, muscle cramps, achy legs, tingling in the face or extremities, dermatitis herpetiformis (painful skin rash or rough texture), mouth sores and mottled tooth discoloration. If you note that you have more than three of these signs or symptoms, it may indicate you have a sensitivity to gluten.

Gluten Sensitivity, Chronic Inflammation, and Bone Loss

Most people assume that if they do not have gastrointestinal signs or symptoms, their bone loss cannot be connected to gluten sensitivity. I certainly held that assumption until only six years ago. I couldn't have been more wrong. I was on my fracturing streak, probably the eighth or ninth of a total of twelve fractured bones, when I was tested for celiac disease. I remember being excited about the possibility of discovering the cause of my osteoporosis. When the results came back negative, I was extremely disappointed. Oh, how I wanted to have celiac disease. A gluten-free diet would have been such an easy solution to my osteoporosis.

Unfortunately, the doctor's interpretation of the lab tests was not completely accurate. He meant well and was trying to help me, but he went by the numbers and assumed that the "negative" on the lab sheet meant that gluten had nothing to do with my bone loss. But, as we are now beginning to realize, negative for celiac disease and negative for gluten sensitivity are two distinctly separate entities. You can test negative for celiac disease and still have gluten as a source of your bone loss. Allow me to explain.

Gluten sensitivity causes bone loss in two ways. The first is obvious. Destruction of the mucosal villi leads to malabsorption and to a deficiency in the prime nutrients for bone. The second cause of bone loss, according to Dr. Daniel Bikle, from the Department of Medicine at the University of California, results from a systemic increase in pro-inflammatory cytokines (2007). When the mucosal cells release zonulin in response to gluten, the tight junctions separate; this creates a leaky gut. Gluten and other food molecules enter through the gut wall and set off an inflammatory response. What you must understand is that sensitivity to gluten, regardless of whether you have been diagnosed with celiac disease, can increase the systemic level of your pro-inflammatory cytokines and contribute to your bone loss.

When the intestinal mucosa becomes inflamed from gluten, the response is maintained by pro-inflammatory cytokines and the activation of NF-KB and T cells (Helms 2005). Of course, you now know that this increases RANKL and is the reason for the accelerated bone loss seen in people with celiac disease (Taranta et al. 2004). And remember, this RANKL connection to gluten and bone loss exists not just in people with gastrointestinal involvement but also in those who have no symptoms at all.

And this is where it gets really interesting. If your intestinal cells already have some degree of leakage from dysbiosis and elevated zonulin, gluten will have easy access through the now not-so-tight, tight junctions. When the large gluten molecules get sucked into places they don't belong, they activate an immune response making you sensitive to gluten. This can happen even though your blood tests or a biopsy reads negative for celiac disease.

If this is happening in your gut, every time you ingest gluten you add fuel to your overall systemic inflammatory load. The amount of gluten consumed is not the important factor; it's your body's sensitivity and its inflammatory response that matter. If you have intestinal permeability and you're sensitive to gluten, you must eliminate it from your diet. Yes, even if your tests show that you have a sensitivity below that necessary for a diagnosis of celiac disease, you should eliminate gluten from your diet.

Diagnosing Gluten Sensitivity

I wish I could tell you that there is a definitive test for gluten sensitivity. Unfortunately, I can't. The gluten protein found in grain is complex and actually takes on different forms, making it difficult to evaluate. What doctors test for is *gliadin,* the component of gluten that typically causes the greatest reactions. But there are other components and forms of gluten and a multitude of ways that your body can react to them. Gluten sensitivity doesn't always involve a reaction within the GI tract. Avoiding gluten-containing grains and watching for changes in signs or symptoms is the best test we have for gluten sensitivity. But if you have no signs or symptoms other than bone loss, this is impractical. You can't wait for two years for your next DXA evaluation to see if your bone density has improved. Currently, the best we can do is to assess gluten sensitivity through intestinal biopsy, blood testing for antibodies, or blood testing for genetic markers.

INTESTINAL BIOPSY

The gold standard for diagnosing celiac disease is to have a biopsy done of your intestinal mucosa. This minimally invasive procedure requires a long flexible tube (endoscope) to be inserted through your mouth and guided into the upper portion of your small intestine (duodenum). Samples of the mucosal wall are retrieved and analyzed. In most cases, cell damage from gluten is concentrated in the upper portion of the intestine, which is where the biopsy sample is taken from. But if the damage is further down in the intestine, the doctor won't be able to see it—and a false negative diagnosis may be made.

ANTIBODIES

There are three commonly used blood tests to check for gluten sensitivity. The first is tissue transglutaminase (tTG) IgA. If you're sensitive to gluten, your immune system will produce antibodies, or immunoglobulins (Ig), to an enzyme called *transglutaminase*, which is produced by the gut to digest gluten. The problem with this is that these antibodies don't just destroy the enzymes; they also destroy the transglutaminase-producing mucosal cells (thus the villi atrophy).

If the results of the tTG blood test are positive, there's a good chance that you are sensitive to gluten, but it is not a definitive test for celiac disease. This is because other immune conditions can also elevate this antibody and create a false-positive test result. Not only that, if mucosal damage is minimal or if your body is functionally unable to produce IgA antibodies, then the tTG test result can be false negative. If you're going to have a tTG test, make sure that your doctor requests a tag-along test called *total IgA*. This is to ensure that you indeed have the capacity to make IgA antibodies; it will rule out any false-negative test result for the tTG.

■ *Celiac Disease and the tTG Test*

When I was tested for celiac disease with the tTG test, the results were interpreted as negative. About a year later, I stumbled on research literature indicating that antibody testing and gluten's relationship to bone loss may not be as simple as a yes-or-no diagnosis for celiac disease. So I immediately looked up my old medical records and realized that gluten just might be a factor in my bone loss after all.

My tTG was negative for celiac disease, but it was measured at 24 EU/ ml, with the reference range set at 25 EU/ml or greater for it to be positive for celiac disease. At 24, it was designated as borderline, only one measly point away from being positive, yet the doctor had diagnosed me as negative for celiac disease and closed the book on this extremely important piece of information.

Remember when I mentioned that the true test for gluten sensitivity is to try a gluten-free diet and see whether a change in signs or symptoms results? When I finally put two and two together, it made sense for me to try a gluten-free diet. But with no obvious gut problems, I didn't really know what to look for. Luckily (I guess you could say that) I did have one thing that I could use as a sign—a very high NTX.

When I had started my own treatment regime for osteoporosis, I was rapidly losing bone. My NTX was 127 nmol, with normal being less than 70 nmol. I had already lowered my NTX into the mid-60s by means of an impeccable diet and supplemental antioxidants, such as alpha-lipoic acid. But I thought I could lower it even further. Endocrinologists are always hoping to get NTX levels into the 30s with bisphosphonates, so it seemed possible that I could get mine a little lower, but without drugs. When I went on a gluten-free diet, my NTX plummeted to 48 nmol and held steady in the high 40s after that.

Whether or not I have celiac disease is still in question. I never did have a small bowel biopsy, but gluten was clearly responsible for at least part of my osteoporosis. My severe bone loss was probably the result of a double insult: chronic inflammation from years of intense physical activity with insufficient nutritional support and a sensitivity to gluten. This double whammy had completely roasted my bones.

The second and third blood tests for gluten sensitivity should always accompany tTG testing. If you are sensitive to gluten, your body will produce antibodies called *antigliadin antibodies* (AGA) as a way to try to destroy this grain protein. AGA comes in two forms: IgA and immuno-globulin (IgG) (thus the two tests). When both forms are positive, you are definitely sensitive to gluten. If just the IgG is elevated and the IgA is normal, that could mean your gut wall is so damaged that you have intestinal permeability (leaky gut). In this case, your reaction to gluten may be because your gut has been so damaged that your immune system is reacting to everything. If this is so, you may be experiencing allergic symptoms to many different foods.

In summary, the tTG will tell you if the villi of your mucosal cells are being damaged, and the two AGA tests will tell you if gluten is the damaging agent. This is why it is important to do all three tests. Recently, a new form of AGA testing has been developed. This is called deamidated gliadin antibody testing, and it appears to have improved accuracy. When being tested for celiac disease, make sure to ask your doctor to use a lab that does deamidated AGA testing.

If you suspect that you have an intolerance to gluten but your antibody tests were inconclusive, you should probably have a biopsy. Additionally, if your bone resorption marker is elevated, try a six-month gluten-free trial and then repeat the bone resorption test. You may be surprised to see a substantially lower score.

GENETIC TESTING

Genetic DNA testing for susceptibility to celiac disease is readily available. Cell samples for the test can either be from blood or a gentle scraping of the cells lining the inside of your mouth. Genetic testing can be especially helpful if you have a close relative with celiac disease but you yourself have no signs or symptoms. Celiac disease is associated with two WBC antigens called HLA-DQ2 and HLA-DQ8. When one or both of these tests is positive, it does not indicate that you have celiac disease. It only means that you have the genes that make you susceptible to the disease. This can be important for you or your family members who may not currently show any signs or symptoms that are reactions to gluten, but would benefit from a gluten-free diet by preventing future gluten-related disease such as osteoporosis.

Treatment for Gluten Sensitivity

If you have celiac disease or are sensitive to gluten, the treatment is simple. Avoid gluten. Wheat, barley, and rye should be eliminated from your diet. Replace them with grains such as teff, quinoa, and buckwheat, which also have the added benefit of being good sources of calcium. For baking, use gluten-free flour made from garbanzo beans, a good source of phytoestrogens and calcium. Many foods contain hidden sources of gluten, so it's wise to invest in a good book on how to eat a gluten-free diet. Note that although, technically, oats do not contain gluten, they are often stored in common granaries and processed on the same machinery as other grains that do contain gluten. This causes the oats to become contaminated with a fine dusting of gluten. Oats should therefore be avoided unless you purchase certified gluten-free oats, which are now becoming readily available.a

Although no medications to treat celiac disease are currently on the market, enzyme proteases are available in supplemental form that can be taken with each meal to help digest small amounts of "hidden gluten" in foods (Cerf-Bensussan et al. 2007). These enzymes are helpful, but for someone with celiac disease, they are not to be used as a substitute for a gluten-free diet. In addition to protease enzymes, there are medications currently undergoing clinical trials. For example, larazotide acetate (AT-1001) helps to inhibit the release of zonulin, therefore reducing mucosal cell disruption, gut inflammation, and the symptoms caused by gluten-containing foods (Paterson et al. 2007).

■ *Mr. Shea's Osteoporosis*

Mr. Shea is a sixty-four-year-old mathematics professor. His doctor referred him to my office for evaluation and nutritional support for a diagnosis of osteoporosis (spine T score -4.4, hips -2.8). Mr. Shea's sedentary lifestyle, struggle with depression, and poor eating habits (high in refined carbohydrates and low in protein) were all risk factors for osteoporosis. He told me that he had never sustained a fracture—at least none that he knew of.

At five feet, eleven inches, Mr. Shea weighed in at 158 pounds. His general demeanor was subdued. He had slight periodontal disease and numerous amalgam-filled cavities, a potential source of mercury toxicity. Mr. Shea's poorly developed muscles felt flabby and had no tone. Moreover, he had a small paunch around his middle and his posture was stooped. These were signs of muscular wasting. His rounded upper back made me suspect osteoporosis-related spinal compression fractures, even though he had no complaints of back pain. Silent vertebral fractures are common with osteoporosis.

Although he did consume dairy products daily, Mr. Shea's diet was poor. His fruit and vegetable intake was minimal. He complained of persistent fatigue and had no sex drive. "I don't drink that much water," he said, "but I have to get up two to three times a night to urinate." This had been going on for at least twenty years. He had no gastrointestinal signs or symptoms.

Mr. Shea's DXA and Laboratory Evaluation

After examining Mr. Shea, I looked over his prior lab tests and then referred him for more testing. I also ordered a set of spinal X-rays.

MR. SHEA'S THORACIC AND LUMBAR SPINE X-RAY RESULTS

The X-rays of Mr. Shea's lumbar (lower) spine showed mild degenerative joint disease and soft-tissue calcifications, but otherwise they were normal. Unfortunately, the X-rays of his thoracic (middle) spine, where his back took a sharp curve forward, disclosed two wedged-shaped compression-type vertebral fractures. Because of these fractures and his extremely low bone density, Mr. Shea needed to be referred to an endocrinologist who specialized in osteoporosis. Not only was it important to rule out other diseases that could be causing secondary osteoporosis, I also felt strongly that Mr. Shea needed to be on an osteoporosis medication. Putting him on a nutritional program would help him enormously in the long run, but for the short term he needed something that would quickly reduce his risk for further fracture.

MR. SHEA'S PRIOR LABORATORY TEST RESULTS

Prior to my first meeting with Mr. Shea, his medical doctor had ordered these tests: a comprehensive metabolic panel (CMP); a complete blood count (CBC); a vitamin D [25(OH)D] test; and serum testosterone. Results from Mr. Shea's CMP showed that he had borderline low blood calcium. This indicated either a scarcity of dietary calcium or magnesium, or a problem with absorption. Also, Mr. Shea's CBC indicated borderline anemia, and his test for vitamin D showed that he was deficient in that vitamin. It's not that uncommon to be low in vitamin D, but when it's coupled with anemia and low blood calcium, that's a fairly sure sign of malabsorption.

The final test that Mr. Shea's doctor had ordered was serum testosterone. Low bone mineral density in men is often correlated to low testosterone, and Mr. Shea's symptom of a nonexistent sex drive strongly suggested low testosterone. Surprisingly though, his test came back quite normal. Mr. Shea's bone loss was beginning to look like a case of malabsorption and chronic inflammation. But I needed a little more information.

To complete Mr. Shea's basic core tests, I ordered a urine calcium test, a celiac profile, and an N-telopeptide (NTX) test. I also gave him a roll of litmus paper and explained how to measure his morning urine pH. In addition, I ordered tests for the inflammation biomarker hs-CRP, the oxidative stress marker 8OH2dG, and because of his sarcopenia (muscle wasting) and depressed demeanor, I ordered a test for the hormone insulin-like growth factor 1 (IGF-1).

When Mr. Shea returned for his follow-up visit two weeks later, we went over his lab results and then filled out his therapeutic targets form.

Mr. Shea's Assessment and Treatment

My initial suspicion that Mr. Shea's bone loss was secondary to a malabsorption disorder did not test out as definitively as I had expected. His results from the celiac profile were interpreted as negative. His tissue transglutaminase (tTG) was elevated, but only to 17 EU/ml, not quite to the antibody reference range level of 19 EU/ml considered necessary for at least a borderline diagnosis of celiac disease. His AGA antibodies were also elevated, but again, not drastically. Mr. Shea did not have celiac disease. But when a person is as osteoporotic as he was and has any sensitivity to gluten, there is only one way to go—get him off gluten!

I didn't even order a biopsy for Mr. Shea. It wouldn't have mattered to me if it came back positive or negative; his antibody level showed clear signs of gluten sensitivity, and with his severe bone loss it was clear that he should eliminate gluten from his diet. Mr. Shea was also sarcopenic, he was depressed, and he was experiencing significant fatigue—all symptoms indicative of systemic inflammation. His physiology was clearly catabolic, so it wasn't a surprise to see his IGF-1 so low. We needed to reduce his inflammation and get him off gluten.

By improving his diet and eliminating gluten, Mr. Shea began to have more energy. He also began to heavily supplement his diet with vitamins, minerals, protein, and essential fatty acids. But good nutrition alone does not—cannot—resolve long-standing deficiency quickly. It would take months, if not years, to fill his reserves.

Central to Mr. Shea's dietary supplementation were not only 1,200 mg of calcium and 600 mg of magnesium, but also vitamins D and K. I started him on 4,000 IU per day of vitamin D_3 and 3 mg per day of vitamin K (K_1 and K_2 MK-4 and MK-7). He continued on this dosage of vitamin D for two months before lowering it to 2,000 IU per day. I wanted to be sure that his vitamin D was at an optimal level not just to improve his bone density, but also because insufficient vitamin D causes muscle weakness (Heaney 2003). Mr. Shea's muscles were already wasting away, and because of his sedentary lifestyle I knew his strength and coordination were poor. He didn't need to compound his risk of falling and breaking a bone due to having low vitamin D. This was easy to correct with supplementation.

To reduce Mr. Shea's inflammation (indicated by the biomarker of elevated hs-CRP) and oxidative stress (8OH2dG), we added fish oil (3g/day), curcumin (400 mg/day), milk thistle (300 mg/day), vitamin C (1,000 mg/day), vitamin E (400 IU/day), N-acetyl cysteine (3,000 mg/day), alpha-lipoic acid (400 mg/day), and taurine (3 g/day). I also included probiotics of live *Lactobacillus* and *Bifidobacterium* cultures (20 billion/day) to improve the health of his gut.

I followed Mr. Shea closely over the next year. We improved his muscle mass, strength, and coordination by persuading him to go to the gym four days a week. We supplemented his diet with DHEA (25 mg/day), whey protein, and an amino acid blend with extra creatine to help increase his IGF-1 and to build muscle mass. We also supplemented his diet with acetyl-L-carnitine to energize his muscles and 200 mcg per day of selenium to help protect his muscles from oxidative damage that can cause sarcopenia (Lauretani et al. 2007). Note: When taking selenium, always ensure a source of iodine (150 mcg/day) to balance selenium's effects on the thyroid gland.

The combination of exercise, diet changes, antioxidants, anabolic nutrition, and his strong desire to regain his health brought Mr. Shea's NTX down to 64 nmol and his IGF-1 up to 93 ng/ml within three months. Although he was improving, the severity of Mr. Shea's bone loss made me insist that he keep his appointment with the endocrinologist. Mr. Shea was prescribed teriparatide (Forteo), the anabolic osteoporosis medication that has had success increasing BMD in cases of severe osteoporosis. After one year of therapy, Mr. Shea's spine T score improved to -3.8 and his hips to -2.6. He was headed in the right direction and no bones were breaking.

LACTOSE INTOLERANCE

The inability to effectively digest lactose, the natural sugar within milk, is called lactose intolerance. This condition often leads to abdominal pain, gas, bloating, and diarrhea when milk products are ingested. In its less severe form, it is referred to as lactase deficiency and may exhibit no symptoms at all. Both conditions are caused by a shortage in the production of the digestive enzyme lactase. This enzyme breaks down lactose into smaller sugar molecules that can readily be absorbed into the bloodstream. When the lactase enzyme is deficient, lactose sits and ferments in the gut, providing a virtual banquet for hungry gut bacteria.

Don't confuse lactose intolerance with an allergy to milk. Lactose intolerance is caused by the deficiency of an enzyme needed to digest the sugar in milk, whereas a milk allergy results from an immune reaction to the proteins found in milk. The two most abundant proteins in milk are casein and whey. Although casein is the most allergenic, whey contains alpha-lactalbumin and beta-lactoglobulin, which may also cause allergic responses. Both conditions can cause abdominal pain, gas, bloating, and diarrhea. But milk allergy, unlike lactose intolerance, may exhibit such signs or symptoms as skin rashes, runny nose, ear infections, eczema, and black rings around the eyes (allergic shiners).

Lactose Intolerance and Bone Loss

As with gluten sensitivity, lactose intolerance can also affect skeletal health adversely. To reduce digestive distress, people who suffer from lactose intolerance often avoid calcium-rich dairy products. This, of course, dramatically reduces their calcium intake. But the low bone density seen in people with lactose intolerance is not all due to insufficient dietary calcium. Research led by Dr. Barbara Obermayer-Pietsch (2007) of the Medical University of Graz, Austria, showed that lactose intolerance actually impairs calcium absorption. Also, undigested lactose alters the pH of the digestive tract, which leads to bacterial overgrowth and, you guessed it, inflammation. This, of course, becomes a chronic source of pro-inflammatory cytokines and systemic inflammation if the person continues to consume dairy products.

CAUSES OF LACTOSE INTOLERANCE

Children can be born lactose intolerant, but this is fairly rare. More commonly, we either see a gradual age-related decline in a person's ability to digest lactose or a more abrupt, genetically determined loss of lactase production from a condition called *adult-type hypolactasia*. Lactose intolerance can also develop as a result of long-standing gut irritation. GI disorders such as irritable bowel and gluten intolerance or parasitic infections such as giardia often lead to intestinal permeability, which then reduces lactase production and creates intolerance to lactose.

TESTING FOR LACTOSE INTOLERANCE

Lactose intolerance is easily identified by simply avoiding dairy products for two weeks, monitoring your signs and symptoms, and then drinking milk. If your symptoms return, it's a good indication that you're lactose intolerant. To differentiate lactose intolerance from an allergic response, your doctor may have to order one of the following two tests.

Lactose tolerance test. For this test, you will be required to ingest a lactose-laden drink and then have several blood draws over the next two hours. If you are unable to digest lactose, your blood glucose level, which should ordinarily rise, will remain steady.

Hydrogen breath test. If you're unable to digest lactose, bacteria will cause it to ferment, which releases hydrogen gas. The gas is absorbed into the bloodstream, carried to your lungs, and then released through capillaries as you exhale. The level of hydrogen in your breath can then be measured.

The Importance of Alternative Calcium Sources

People with osteoporosis often feel pressured to eat dairy products, even if they're lactose intolerant. I can't tell you how many times I've been asked, "But don't you eat dairy?" If you don't produce enough lactase, and 60 to 70 percent of adults don't, then you should consider excluding dairy from your diet. A recent study (Obermayer-Pietsch et al. 2007) concluded that individuals with adult-type hypolactasia should eliminate even hidden sources of lactose, such as those found in processed meats, bread, cakes, and drinks, because even small amounts can interfere with the absorption of calcium. If you're lactose intolerant, you should read the labels on food products.

Although some lactose-sensitive people can tolerate yogurt because its bacteria culture produces some lactase, you'll still need to find alternative sources of calcium if you eliminate dairy from your diet. Eat more high-calcium foods such as kale, broccoli, bok choy, sardines, and soy milk. We're fortunate because many foods are now fortified with calcium. But even with all of these great sources, if you are lactose intolerant and avoiding dairy products, you'll need to supplement your diet with calcium.

PUTTING IT ALL TOGETHER

Reducing GI distress increases nutrient absorption and eliminates an insidious source of systemic inflammation. Whether the distress is due to impaired HCl production, gut dysbiosis, intestinal parasites, gluten sensitivity, lactose intolerance, or any other GI disturbance, if you are going to improve your skeletal health, you will first need to ensure the health of your gut. Make sure to ask your doctor for a food allergy or intolerance assessment if you're experiencing any abdominal-related signs or symptoms or even unexplained depression, brain fog, hyperactivity, headaches, chronic mucous congestion, recurrent sinus infections, ear infections, sore throat, rashes, fatigue, or joint or muscle pains.

Food Sensitivity Testing

Improving gut function begins with identifying the irritants that are causing you harm. The three best tools for doing this are an elimination diet, food antibody testing, and a stool analysis.

ELIMINATION DIET

Foods that irritate your body can be identified through an elimination diet. You do this by temporarily excluding all common dietary triggers of inflammation, and then reintroducing them one by one into your diet. The exclusion period usually lasts two to four weeks, during which time all foods that contain common allergens, such as the gluten-containing grains (wheat, barley, and rye), dairy, eggs, corn, white potatoes, tomatoes, peas, beans, soy, nuts, peanuts, shellfish, citrus fruits, and refined sugars, are avoided.

This sounds like just about everything but, believe it or not, there is a lot more out there to eat. Lamb, fish, poultry, nongluten grains (such as rice and quinoa), sweet potatoes, noncitrus fruits, and vegetables (except those listed above) are all foods that you can chow down on. The important part of this test is to be sure to write down the date when you reintroduce a food, and then to record any symptomatic reactions that develop. Make sure to wait two to three days before reintroducing the next food item. Although an elimination diet is best undertaken with the supervision of your health care provider, there are certainly many written sources to help guide you.

FOOD ANTIBODY TESTING

For many years, testing for food and environmental allergens was done primarily by scratching the surface of the skin with an allergen and then observing the response. But the reaction to a food at the surface of your skin can differ hugely from the reaction as it passes through the gut. For that reason, food allergy testing is more helpful when done through a blood test evaluation of the IgE and IgG antibodies.

Adverse reactions to food can be immediate or delayed. A severe, immediate immune response, such as difficulty breathing after ingesting peanuts or explosive diarrhea after drinking milk, is mediated by IgE (you can think of it as E for emergency) antibodies. Most food allergy testing is traditionally done by testing for IgE antibodies. However, there is another type of antibody testing, called IgG (think of G for general or gradual). *IgG testing* identifies delayed reactions that are typically less severe but are still a source of ill health.

When someone has multiple IgG food sensitivities, it can be a sign of intestinal permeability and a major source of chronic inflammation. IgG testing can vary in accuracy depending on the expertise of the laboratory performing the analysis. Because of this, use IgG testing with some caution. This type of testing is best used as a guide to improve your health and not as firm documentation of any food sensitivity you may have.

STOOL ANALYSIS

When I send in a stool sample to the lab, I always feel some sympathy for the poor technician who has to look at it. But when the results return, my feelings of guilt quickly vanish. Chronic digestive problems in my patients with osteoporosis are extremely common, and by analyzing their stool we often identify a problem that needs to be corrected. My objective is to optimize a patient's ability to absorb nutrients and to eliminate any unnecessary sources of chronic inflammation. When the lab results show undigested food in the patient's stool, abnormal pH, elevated inflammatory markers, parasites, or an overgrowth of bacteria or yeast, we can correct these problems and the patient's health improves.

If you suspect that you have a gut dysfunction, ask your doctor about a stool analysis. The specialty labs listed in the Resources section will be your best sources for high-quality stool analysis testing. A stool analysis is useful for determining whether your gut is a gateway to health or a road to bone loss.

Repairing Your Gut

Normalizing gut health is accomplished by following the 4R program. This refers to a therapeutic program for the GI tract that was originally developed by Jeffery Bland, Ph.D. It includes the following four basic steps: remove, replace, reinoculate, and repair (Lukaczer 2006).

Remove. The first step for correcting any GI disorder is to remove the irritant. This may be as simple as eliminating gluten or a specific food from your diet. It may also require treatment to eliminate gut pathogens (such as bacteria, yeast, or parasites) through the use of antimicrobial, antifungal, or antiparasitic herbs or medications.

Replace. The second step is to replace hydrochloric acid or digestive enzymes if they are not being produced in the amount necessary to achieve optimal digestion and gut health.

Reinoculate. Whether a GI problem is based in the overabundance of a pathogen or a scarcity of one or more of the normally occurring, or commensal, species of the gut, the result can often be the same: intestinal permeability and ill health. By reinoculating the gut, that is, by reintroducing live cultures of microorganisms called *probiotics,* which consist of the *Lactobacillus, Bifidobacterium*, and *Saccharomyces* genuses, it is possible to prevent recolonization by pathogens and other opportunistic species. Moreover, the use of a *pre*biotic, such as psyllium fiber, arabinogalactan (an immune-stimulating dietary fiber made from larch wood), or a simple plant sugar such as inulin, will help to promote the growth of good microbes.

Probiotics stimulate toll-like receptors and promote oral tolerance by muting their immune response. It's important to understand that reinoculation does not shift into automatic gear after a few weeks of taking high doses of probiotics; continued daily administration is required. Once a GI tract has become dysbiotic, it has a tendency to revert back to microbial imbalance even after it has been successfully treated. Therefore, probiotics should not be completely discontinued after the initial treatment phase. Continued intake of a lower daily dosage, usually 3 to 10 billion, should be maintained. The oral tolerance maintained by this ongoing daily supplementation will help to mute the immunological response to harmless bacteria and food particles, reduce T cell activation, and limit the production of pro-inflammatory cytokines and RANKL.

Repair. The final step in the 4R program is to repair the gut. This is accomplished by providing nutrition that specifically supports the regeneration of gut tissues. Fish oil (for essential fatty acids), zinc, manganese, pantothenic acid (vitamin B_5), vitamin D, fiber, and the antioxidant vitamins A, C, E, and beta-carotene are all important for the repair of the gut wall. But the most important nutritional supplement that you can take for gut repair is L-glutamine. This amino acid serves as fuel for intestinal cells and is essential for maintaining gut health. Quan et al. (2004) demonstrated that glutamine not only helps to repair the gut and reduce intestinal permeability, it also reduces gastrointestinal inflammation.

CHAPTER SIX

Your Body's Regulatory Hormones: The Pulse of Skeletal Health

Maintaining the correct mineral balances within your blood while simultaneously preserving your bone strength is a difficult feat that demands not just a healthy diet, but energetic hormones too. Your body's hormonal flows are comparable to the water supply in a forest. Its rivers, creeks, ponds, and underground springs, and even its moist, atmospheric breath, intermingle to generate a precarious balance of growth, senescence, death, and rebirth. The seasons charge this watery network with an undulating pulse that surges throughout the forest as through a single organism. In your body, the ebbs and flows of regulatory hormones manage a similarly delicate balance.

Hormones are naturally produced chemicals. They are formed within your various organs and secreted into the bloodstream, where they carry messages from one gland or organ system to another. The major hormone-producing organs are the pituitary, pineal, thymus, thyroid, parathyroids, adrenals, pancreas, ovaries, testes, and yes, the skeleton. The hormones secreted by these organs are so powerful that just a small variation one way or the other can be the difference between health and disease. Having just the right amounts is crucial for maintaining normal physiological function, including the mineral balance of your skeleton.

Your body produces two general types of hormones: steroid and peptide. *Steroid hormones* are made from cholesterol in your adrenal glands and ovaries or testes. They act mainly to regulate sexual maturation and fertility. These are often referred to as the "raging hormones" of teenagers.

The less sexy *peptide hormones* are made from amino acids, the building blocks of protein. These act to regulate energy balance, sleep cycles, mineral and electrolyte levels, and other mechanisms of metabolism.

If you have osteoporosis, there's a good chance that the flow of one or more of your hormones is out of kilter. Trying to maintain skeletal balance without normal hormonal levels is like sowing seed on dry, barren land and hoping for a forest to grow. Without the flow of water through the land, or hormones through your body, the impulse for growth is missing. The hormonal flow is strong when you're young, but as you age or fall into ill health, hormone production wanes and this can weaken bones. Not just aging leads to reduced hormone production. Chronic inflammation, gastrointestinal dysfunction, emotional or physical distress, and chronic exposure to toxins all lead to reduced hormone production. These all conspire against hormone production, and they're all conditions that can be corrected.

When, through good nutrition and balanced lifestyle, you are able to reduce inflammation, improve gut function, and cleanse toxins from your system, your hormone production will improve. Often this is all that is necessary to rectify hormonal imbalances. But if your efforts fail and levels remain inadequate, you might choose to replenish key hormones with the use of medications or biologically identical hormones.

What follows is an explanation of the three major groups of hormones that support bone mineral maintenance. Those that regulate calcium and bone mineral equilibrium comprise the first group. They are parathyroid hormone (PTH), calcitriol (the hormonal form of vitamin D), and calcitonin. Each can be supplied from outside sources if necessary.

The second group is composed of three sex hormones: estrogen and progesterone (the "female" hormones) and testosterone (the "male" hormone). When necessary, these can be restored to optimal levels by the use of biologically identical hormones.

The final group of hormones is necessary for maintaining growth and metabolic balance. These are insulin-like growth factor 1 (IGF-1), dehydroepiandrosterone (DHEA), cortisol, thyroid hormone, osteocalcin, serotonin, and melatonin.

CALCIUM-REGULATING HORMONES

If calcium intake is insufficient, its blood levels will fall and your body will respond by releasing three different hormones. *Parathyroid hormone* taps the mineral reserves in bone by stimulating osteoclastic activity to increase bone resorption. At the same time, vitamin D from both exposure to sunlight and dietary sources is activated within the kidneys to form calcitriol, the activated form of vitamin D, which then acts to increase calcium absorption within the small intestine. Once normal blood calcium levels have been regained, the hormone calcitonin is then released from the thyroid gland to dampen PTH-induced osteoclastic activity. This hormonal feedback loop ensures the integrity of bone's mineral reserves.

Parathyroid Hormone

When blood calcium is low, sensors in four small glands situated on either side of the thyroid gland in your neck immediately signal for the release of parathyroid hormone (PTH). When calcium levels drop, PTH acts to rectify the problem in three ways: First, it limits kidney excretion of calcium through the urine. Second, PTH activates vitamin D, which leads to increased absorption of calcium from food. And finally, PTH stimulates bone cells (both the osteoclasts and osteoblasts) to increase bone remodeling, an action that initiates the release of calcium into the bloodstream. Together, these actions on the kidneys, intestines, and skeleton are what make PTH the primary regulator of blood calcium levels.

A manufactured form of PTH called teriparatide (Forteo) is available to treat severe osteoporosis. When a small amount of this medication is injected under the skin on a daily basis, it acts not to tear down bone (as might be expected from PTH) but to stimulate bone formation. This medication can be extremely effective both in building bone and in reducing fractures.

Calcitriol

Adequate vitamin D is necessary for the absorption of calcium and to stimulate osteoblasts to form bone. It also helps to maintain blood calcium levels for normal heart, nerve, and muscle functioning. You obtain this vitamin either through the conversion of a cholesterol-based substance in the skin during sunlight exposure or through your diet. Whether through sun exposure or diet, the vitamin D is then converted in the liver to its storage form, 25-hydroxy vitamin D [25(OH)D] or *cholecalciferol*. When needed, PTH converts this inactive form in the kidneys into *calcitriol*, or 1,25-dihydroxy vitamin D [$1,25(OH)_2D$], which is considered the active, hormonal form of this vitamin. Calcitriol increases intestinal absorption of calcium, and when the correct balance of blood calcium levels is restored, it then acts as a feedback mechanism to signal the parathyroid glands to stop releasing PTH.

This is where things get a little complicated. Calcitriol levels often remain normal even when you are deficient in inactive vitamin D. It's only when inactive vitamin D is abysmally low that calcitriol levels will also be low. With inadequate vitamin D, your body continues to stimulate the release of PTH to break down more bone for its calcium. Dr. Michael Holick and coleagues (2005), at the Boston University School of Medicine, found that 52 percent of postmenopausal women with osteoporosis had inadequate vitamin D levels. This is why it's so important to make sure your doctor measures the storage (inactive) form of vitamin D. He or she may also choose to test calcitriol, but this is necessary only under certain circumstances.

The level of vitamin D in your blood should be maintained at between 35 ng/ml and 80 ng/ml. Sunlight, ten to fifteen minutes a day, three to four days a week, will help keep your D levels optimal. Sorry, but if you live north of Georgia, you get absolutely no vitamin D from the sun in the winter—even if you sunbathe naked and shivering all day long. Fatty fish such as salmon provide some vitamin D, but even this source has its problems. Wild-caught fish often contain unacceptable amounts of mercury, and farm-raised salmon have only 10 to 25 percent of the vitamin D of wild salmon. It's therefore safest to supplement with 2,000 IU per day of vitamin D while still including some fish in your diet.

If you are extremely low in vitamin D, your doctor may prescribe a large dose (up to 50,000 IU/week) of vitamin D_2, which is called *ergocalciferol*. This form of vitamin D is synthetic and different from natural vitamin D_3. Not only is synthetic D_2 different than the vitamin D produced by your body, it also has less biological function. When my patients are severely low in vitamin D, I have them take 4,000 IU per day of vitamin D_3 for two months, and then I recheck their blood level. If their vitamin D level has increased sufficiently, they can then be reduced to 2,000 IU per day. Because vitamin D is a fat-soluble vitamin, it can be stored in the body, and therefore it has the potential for toxicity. For this reason, you would not want to exceed 2,000 IU per day for an extended period unless under the direction of a physician.

Calcitonin

Calcitonin tempers the effects of PTH. Secreted by the thyroid gland, calcitonin promotes the transfer of calcium to bone by inhibiting osteoclastic resorption. When blood calcium is too low, PTH acts to release calcium from bone by stimulating osteoclasts to speed up resorption. As blood calcium rises, special sensors in the thyroid gland react by stimulating the release of calcitonin. This amazing hormone has the ability to shrink osteoclasts and disempower them. The result is to lower blood calcium levels. Seesawing back and forth, minute changes in PTH, calcitonin, and calcitriol manage blood calcium equilibrium. What a balancing act! Calcitonin nasal spray derived from salmon was one of the first medications developed for the treatment of osteoporosis. Its effect on improving bone mineral density (BMD) is modest, but it does seem to reduce the incidence of vertebral fractures.

SEX HORMONES

Estrogen, progesterone, and testosterone comprise the second group of regulatory hormones. These are all produced by the sex glands. For years, hormone replacement therapy (HRT) in the form of estrogen plus progestin (a synthetic form of progesterone) was the treatment of choice for menopausal symptoms and the prevention of bone loss. This changed in 2002 when the Women's Health Initiative (WHI), a study conducted to determine the risks and benefits of HRT, was prematurely ended after it was found that long-term use of these drugs increased the risk of heart attack, stroke, venous blood clots, and breast cancer. Although it was also determined that HRT decreased osteoporotic fractures and lowered the risk of colon cancer, the study concluded that the risks of hormone therapy outweigh its benefits. This landmark study dramatically reduced the use of HRT for osteoporosis and created a financial windfall for the manufacturers of bisphosphonates, which became the new drug therapy of choice for treating bone loss.

Estrogen

The loss of estrogen increases your risk for osteoporosis. Estrogen's primary role in maintaining skeletal health is not to build bone but, by tempering osteoclastic activity, to prevent its destruction. Although there are three forms of estrogen produced naturally in your body, estrone (E1), estradiol (E2), and estriol (E3), it is *estradiol* from the ovaries that is most vital to skeletal health prior to menopause. Blood levels of estrogen begin to decline five or so years before menopause begins (normally between the ages of forty-eight and fifty). After this time, although fat cells continue to produce significant amounts, estradiol levels are only a fraction of what they were during premenopausal years. After menopause, the adrenal glands produce the less potent *estrone,* which helps maintain (at a reduced level) estrogen activity. This changeover in the predominant estrogen found in the body is often inadequate for maintaining bone density. It's not unusual for bone loss to reach 2 to 4 percent a year during the five to seven years immediately after menopause. This critical period of rapid bone loss is a time of heightened fracture risk, especially in the bones of the forearm and spine.

Estrogen not only limits bone resorption, it also helps increase calcium absorption, stimulates the development of bone-building osteoblasts and, as you learned in chapter 5, helps maintain oral tolerance to minor gut irritants, thereby dampening excessive inflammation. It also promotes bone formation by increasing IGF-1, limits pro-inflammatory cytokines and RANKL, curtails excessive T cell activation, and acts as a switch manager for the differentiation of stem cells into osteoblasts.

EXERCISE 6.1: Signs and Symptoms of Low Estrogen (for Women)

Look at the following list of common signs and symptoms of low estrogen. Highlight or circle any that apply to you. If you check three or more, your estrogen levels are probably too low.

Common signs and symptoms of low estrogen: Hot flashes or night sweats, dry or thin skin, vaginal dryness, painful sexual intercourse, sagging breasts, dry eyes, anxiety or panic attacks, depression, mood swings, frequent urination, memory loss or difficulty concentrating, sleep disturbances, rapid pulse, and atrophic cells on a Pap smear.

SHOULD YOU CONSIDER THE USE OF HRT?

Because of the statistical interpretation of the research obtained from the WHI study, many women, and most doctors, no longer consider the use of HRT an option for reducing bone loss. Currently, HRT for the treatment of osteoporosis without menopausal symptoms is discouraged. However, the WHI study used a standard high dose of 0.625 mg of conjugated equine estrogen (CEE; derived from the urine of pregnant horses) and 2.5 mg of the synthetic progestin, medroxyprogesterone acetate (MPA), from which to draw conclusions. In addition, the women in this study averaged sixty-three years of age, while most women considering HRT are much younger. Furthermore, one-half of the women in this study either smoked or had a history of smoking, and one-third were obese or had high blood pressure (Warren and Halpert 2004).

Smoking and obesity are risk factors for breast cancer, and high blood pressure is a risk for heart disease. So you can see how the interpretation of the WHI study may have lead to erroneous conclusions—an unfortunate research outcome that may, in retrospect, be a great disservice to those women who could benefit from hormone therapy.

If you are osteoporotic and experiencing uncomfortable menopausal symptoms, such as hot flashes, night sweats, or vaginal dryness, talk with your doctor to determine whether HRT is appropriate for you. In the Women's Health, Osteoporosis, Progestin, Estrogen (HOPE) study, it was shown that substantially lower doses (0.45 mg CEE and 0.3 mg MPA) of HRT can have a significant bone-sparing effect (Lindsay et al. 2002).

A review of studies (van de Weijer et al. 2007) concluded that the use of low-dose HRT (0.3 mg CEE and 1.5 mg MPA) to treat women with menopausal symptoms not only had fewer side effects than the standard dosing, it also increased spine and hip bone density and did not appear to carry an increased risk for heart disease, vascular disease, or breast cancer. What may be the most important recent clinical trial (Ettinger et al. 2004) showed that an ultralow dose of 0.014 mg/day transdermal (applied through the skin) estradiol was able to increase BMD.

This tells us that less is better. If you and your doctor determine that you would benefit from HRT, make sure you follow these instructions: First, have your doctor run a test to determine how your body will process estrogen. This is important because, depending on your genetic makeup, you may break down estrogen into more or less harmful substances before they are excreted from your body. Second, use bioidentical hormones (see below). Third, use the least amount of hormone replacement possible.

BIOIDENTICAL HORMONES

Bioidentical hormones are made from plants and are molecularly identical to the estrogens, progesterone, and testosterone that are produced in humans. Because of this, bioidentical hormones can fit exactly into a cell's hormone receptor sites and not cause some of the undesirable side effects seen with the medications used in the WHI study.

The preferred method of administering estrogen is through cream or a patch. This transdermal approach prevents *first-pass metabolism,* where estrogen is converted by the liver into *estrone* (the form of estrogen predominately linked to cancer). Many doctors now combine the estrogens into an E3 and E2 product (80:20 ratio) called *bi-est,* or into an E3, E2, and E1 product (80:10:10 ratio) called *tri-est.* These formulas are ideal for obtaining both estriol's skeletal and cardiovascular benefits and estradiol's effects of relieving menopausal symptoms.

ESTROGEN METABOLISM

After estrogen is used by your body, it is broken down into several metabolites before being excreted. (A *metabolite* is any substance produced by metabolism or a metabolic process.) Two of the most important are 2-hydroxyestrone (2OHE1) and 16-alpha-hydroxyestrone (16αOHE1). 2OHE1 is considered to be beneficial in that it is no longer estrogenically active and therefore won't stimulate cancer growth. On the other hand, 16αOHE1 is much more estrogenically active and has been linked to breast cancer. You don't want to produce a lot of this metabolite and have it hang around in your system for too long before being excreted.

The ratio of these two metabolites in women may be more important than the overall level of estrogen. If the 2OHE1 to 16αOHE1 ratio is too low, there is a greater risk for cancer and other conditions associated with an excess of estrogen. If the ratio is reversed and 2OHE1, the less active metabolite, predominates, there may not be enough estrogen activity. In the latter case you would have an increased risk for osteoporosis (Leelawattana et al. 2000). Your doctor can assess this ratio through a lab test. If the ratio is unfavorable, that gives you two valuable pieces of information: First, it may indicate that you should avoid using HRT altogether. Second, by altering this ratio through nutritional supplements and dietary changes, it can be used as an objective target for reducing your risk of cancer. If you are considering HRT therapy, and even if you are only concerned about breast cancer, this test is highly recommended.

PHYTOESTROGENS

Phytoestrogens (isoflavones and lignans) are plant products with weak estrogenic activity. The best sources are genistein and daidzein from soybeans, as well as garbanzo beans (chickpeas), bean spouts, asparagus, garlic, flaxseed, black cohosh root, and resveratrol from grapes.

These all have beneficial estrogenic effects on bone. A 2006 study of 136 Japanese women demonstrated that a combined regimen of 75 mg per day of isoflavones plus walking three times a week for one year increased BMD (Wu et al. 2006). The authors concluded that isoflavones may be beneficial in preventing osteoporosis.

An article in the *Journal of the American Dietetic Association* (Heaney, Carey, and Harkness 2005) noted that there have been at least sixteen observational studies and ten intervention trials where soy or soy isoflavones have been found to have beneficial effects on bone health. They further state that soy isoflavone doses of 80 to 90 mg per day may be necessary to positively affect bone health.

If you're using soy products for their phytoestrogen effects on bone health, consider supplementing with short-chain fructo-oligosaccharides (SC-FOS). These indigestible sugars appear to help gut microbes convert daidzein (a soy protein) into the active phytoestrogen equol (Mathey et al. 2007). Equol is considered the phytoestrogen mainly responsible for soy's ability to prevent bone loss. Poor gut health and dysbiosis would therefore potentially reduce soy's ability to promote skeletal health. Because soy intake levels necessary to affect bone health are hard to obtain through diet, many people have begun supplementing with soy isoflavones such as *ipriflavone.*

This synthetic form of soy isoflavone is popular for treating osteoporosis. Its effectiveness and safety have recently been challenged in a study published in the *Journal of the American Medical Association*, which failed to show any improvement in bone density and indicated that the use of ipriflavone can result in lymphocytopenia, a reduction in white blood cells (Alexandersen et al. 2001). Further studies are needed to determine the safety of soy isoflavones and their benefits, if any, for the treatment of osteoporosis.

Progesterone

As with estrogen, progesterone in premenopausal women is produced primarily in the ovaries. After menopause, the adrenal glands take on the task. Progesterone is thought to promote skeletal health through two primary mechanisms: First, progesterone receptors have been identified on osteoblasts, indicating that this hormone has a role in stimulating bone collagen formation. And second, progesterone actually may block the adrenal gland hormone cortisol, which is known to have a deleterious effect on bone density.

Progesterone production, like bone density, begins to decline when women are in their thirties. In addition to this natural decline, undue stress and *anovulatory* menstrual cycles (those without ovulation) reduce progesterone levels, contributing to early bone loss. When you're physically or emotionally stressed, the adrenal glands respond by releasing cortisol. Chronically elevated cortisol has negative effects on your health, including a reduction in your ability to make progesterone.

EXERCISE 6.2: Signs and Symptoms of Low Progesterone (for Women)

If you have bone loss, take a look at the following list of signs and symptoms. If you highlight or circle two or more of these symptoms, that may indicate your progesterone production is suboptimal. Your doctor can use laboratory testing to evaluate your ability to produce progesterone.

Signs and symptoms of low progesterone in women: Anxiety, mood swings, sleep disturbances, irritability or being easily startled, depression, and irregular or heavy periods.

If you are considering progesterone hormone therapy, keep in mind there is a difference between synthetic progesterones (progestins), as found in Provera (medroxyprogesterone) and Prempro (conjugated estrogens and medroxyprogesterone), and natural progesterone. Progestins are chemically different than the progesterone you produce in your body, and they increase your risk for breast cancer. Natural progesterone does not carry the same risk and can help to increase your bone density. But remember, estrogen and progesterone work together. You will need to work closely with your doctor to determine which hormone or combination of hormones is appropriate for your specific needs.

Transdermal progesterone creams have become popular, but their use for the treatment of osteoporosis can be problematic due to irregular dosing, and their effectiveness is unproven (Elshafie and Eweis 2007). Oral bioidentical progesterone will ensure exact dosages and may be a better choice. However, if your preference is transdermal application, don't use over-the-counter creams. Make sure your progesterone prescription is filled by a compounding pharmacy.

Testosterone

Although low estrogen is clearly associated with increased fracture risk in both women and men, the effects of testosterone have been less definitive. Low testosterone in men has been definitely linked to low bone density, but when the correlation is made to an increase in fracture risk, it appears that the relationship is due more to the fact that low testosterone causes increased systemic inflammation than from the beneficial effects of the hormone itself. Research (Maggio et al. 2006) has revealed that as men age, their blood levels of the pro-inflammatory cytokine interleukin-6 rise as testosterone levels fall. Low levels of both estrogen and testosterone are known to increase inflammation, and both are linked to osteoporosis in men and women.

The blood level of a protein called sex hormone binding globulin (SHBG) may possibly be more important than either your estrogen or testosterone level. Too little SHBG, and hormone receptors won't be activated (Caldwell et al. 2006); too much, and sex hormones are not freely available to initiate cellular activity. When sex hormones are bound to SHBG, their ability to affect bone and other organs is limited. Your doctor can check the level of SHBG in your blood. If it is abnormally high, make sure to also have your IGF-1 checked. Low IGF-1 will cause SHBG to increase, thus binding and restricting sex hormone activity.

EXERCISE 6.3: Signs and Symptoms of Low Testosterone (for Men)

The following list details the signs and symptoms of low testosterone. Read through the list and highlight or circle any that apply to you. If you check two or more, there is a good chance that your testosterone is too low. But even if you have none of these signs or symptoms and you have osteoporosis, you should make sure that your doctor orders lab tests to evaluate both your testosterone and estrogen levels.

Signs and symptoms of low testosterone in men: Low sex drive, erectile dysfunction, sleep disturbances, loss of muscle mass (lean tissue), fat accumulation around your abdominal area, loss of pubic hair, fatigue or lack of energy, lack of initiative, depression, and irritability.

Due to a heightened risk for prostate cancer, the use of testosterone replacement therapy (TRT) is recommended only for men who have *hypogonadism-related osteoporosis*. This condition results in deficient testosterone production by the testes. If your blood testosterone level is below 300 ng/dl or you have erectile dysfunction, your doctor may want to prescribe a transdermal testosterone patch to help boost your blood levels of this hormone.

HORMONES FOR GROWTH AND METABOLIC BALANCE

The final group of hormones is involved in maintaining the general growth and metabolic balance of your body.

Insulin-like Growth Factor 1

You were introduced to insulin-like growth factor 1 (IGF-1) in chapter 3. IGF-1 is considered to be the most powerful natural anabolic agent in your body. Its production and release from the liver is dependent on good nutrition. Although excess production of IGF-1 is not healthy and can promote cancer growth, deficient levels lead to osteoporosis and poor muscle mass, sarcopenia. (Remember the Tissue Poke exercise in chapter 3?). Chronic inflammation and high levels of the pro-inflammatory cytokine IL-6 cause IGF-1 blood levels to drop.

EXERCISE 6.4: Signs and Symptoms of Low IGF-1

Signs and symptoms of low IGF-1 are not specific and may be similar to those of depression, low testosterone, or hypothyroidism. Nevertheless, read through the following list and highlight or circle those that relate to your situation. If you mark four or more, ask your doctor to test the level of your IGF-1.

Signs and symptoms of low IGF-1: Muscle wasting, fatigue, poor muscle strength, low energy, diminished exercise tolerance, thinning of the skin with very fine wrinkling, skin that "hangs" (like sagging cheeks), depression, difficulty staying up past nine or ten in the evening, sleep disturbances, poor cognition, grumpiness, elevated total cholesterol and triglycerides, low high-density lipoprotein (HDL) cholesterol, and chronic inflammation (check your biomarkers of inflammation).

If you are low in IGF-1, use it as a therapeutic marker and refer back to chapter 3. You will find ways there to increase your production of this important hormone, which will help to improve your muscle mass and skeletal health. Reducing chronic inflammation is central to regaining a healthy level of IGF-1.

DHEA

Dehydroepiandrosterone (DHEA) is the "mother hormone" to estrogen, progesterone, and testosterone. DHEA has long been considered the antiaging hormone. It is naturally produced in your body by the adrenal glands and peaks in production by your midthirties. After this time, your DHEA blood levels slowly decline. That is why this hormone is often viewed as a biomarker for aging. Low DHEA reduces your ability to produce sex hormones and is consistently correlated to chronic diseases, including osteoporosis. In a recent study with elderly men, low DHEA was correlated to hip and arm fractures independent of their BMD (Ohlsson et al. 2007).

There has been considerable research regarding the use of oral DHEA supplementation for treating low bone density. Some studies indicate that there is a benefit to the skeleton from supplementing with DHEA, while others fail to show positive effects. For example, studies with anorexic girls indicate that DHEA lowers bone resorption and increases bone formation (Gordon et al. 1999, 2002). But in a study with middle-aged to elderly men, supplemented with 90 mg per day, there appeared to be no skeletal benefit (Kahn and Halloran 2002). Clearly, the jury is still out as to whether DHEA supplementation is beneficial for skeletal health.

That said, if you're a women with low DHEA (and do not have a hormone-sensitive cancer), supplementing with micronized oral DHEA, 25 to 50 mg per day, may prove beneficial. A brief explanation of postmenopausal estrogen production will help you to understand the logic behind this recommendation.

During menopause, there are some amazing changes that take place in your body. One is that estrogen production switches from the ovaries over to the adrenal glands. When the ovaries stop producing estrogen, systemic levels plummet dramatically. They actually drop to a level below that seen in men. Furthermore, instead of estradiol, it is estrone that becomes the predominant estrogen. Although systemic estrone helps to maintain skeletal health, it is the local production within the skeleton itself that becomes the primary source of estrogen for bone preservation. Also, it is locally within the individual bones that testosterone and DHEA are converted to estrogen by the enzyme aromatase, which is produced by the osteoblasts (Simpson et al. 2005). Without adequate testosterone and DHEA, you will not be able to produce enough estrogen to maintain your bone density.

It turns out that after menopause, your circulating levels of testosterone and DHEA may be more important than your estradiol levels for providing your bones with the estrogen they need to remain strong and healthy.

EXERCISE 6.5:   Signs and Symptoms of Low DHEA

It is not unusual for my patients with very low bone density to have low levels of DHEA. If you highlight or check off three or more of the following signs and symptoms, you may have low levels of DHEA.

Signs and symptoms of low DHEA: Declining health, chronic high feelings of stress, chronic fatigue or low energy, diminished pubic hair, low sex drive, elevated cortisol, low cholesterol, and chronic inflammation (check your biomarkers of inflammation).

If you suspect that your DHEA is low, ask your doctor for a laboratory assessment before beginning to use DHEA supplementation. DHEA is clinically measured in two forms: active DHEA and DHEA-sulfate (DHEA-S), which is its inactive or reserve form. When my female patients have low DHEA, I ask them to supplement with 25 to 50 mg per day of micronized DHEA (which is pulverized into particles that are just a few microns in diameter and therefore more easily assimilated), in addition to 5 g per day of an amino acid blend. For osteoporotic men, I have them take 10 to 50 mg per day of DHEA unless they have a history of an enlarged prostate or prostate cancer. DHEA supplementation is contraindicated with a history of any hormone-sensitive cancer. DHEA should be used only while under the supervision of your doctor.

Depending on your specific situation, your doctor may choose to use *pregnenolone*, the precursor to DHEA, to increase your DHEA levels.

Cortisol

The hormone cortisol is released from the adrenal glands in response to stress. This is the hormone that allows your body to respond to danger immediately. It does this by increasing your blood pressure to enhance muscular power and your blood glucose to provide additional energy. But prolonged elevation of cortisol levels, which happens as a result of chronic stress, increases your risk for disease. Cortisol reduces the ability of your osteoblasts to form bone; it can also throw the switch that diverts the mesenchymal stem cells away from becoming osteoblasts toward becoming fat cells (in the bone marrow) (see chapter 4). It's no wonder that chronic stress and elevated cortisol levels are associated with reduced bone density and elevated fracture risk.

Chronic stress also reduces DHEA levels. This leads to a high ratio of cortisol to DHEA, which lowers IGF-1 and the ability to form bone. The stress of sleep deprivation has been shown to increase cortisol, reduce IGF-1, and lower BMD (Specker et al. 2007).

EXERCISE 6.6: Signs and Symptoms of High Cortisol

Excess production of cortisol can be a sign of serious disease, such as pituitary or adrenal tumors. It may also be due to overactivation of the adrenal glands caused by chronic stress. The following are signs and symptoms of elevated cortisol. If you circle more than three, there is a good possibility that your stress and cortisol levels are chronically excessive.

Signs and symptoms of high cortisol: Irritability, increased blood pressure, elevated cholesterol, irregular or premature loss of menstrual periods, depression, and anorexia nervosa.

When life becomes so stressful that survival, not sex, is the body's main mission, blood cortisol levels skyrocket, while blood levels of the reproductive hormones (estrogen, progesterone, and testosterone) fall. One of the body's mechanisms for bone preservation during limited times of stress is to produce more progesterone, which blocks the damaging effects of cortisol on osteoblasts. But when severe stress becomes chronic, this safety mechanism is dismantled, and the body is thrown into full preservation mode, which both reduces osteoblast cell activation and progesterone production.

In addition to looking at signs and symptoms, you can have your adrenal health assessed by means of a simple salivary cortisol test. If you have elevated cortisol, minimize your stress, get enough rest, and reduce your intake of refined carbohydrates. Since cortisol is a natural anti-inflammatory hormone, if you reduce the inflammation in your body, you will also lower your cortisol. Because gastrointestinal dysfunction is a common source of systemic inflammation, if you eliminate allergy-producing foods and normalize your gut's microflora, you will lower your cortisol levels. Supplementation with vitamin D and botanicals such as ginseng and licorice can also help lower cortisol.

Thyroid Hormone

The thyroid gland, situated next to the voice box in your neck, produces thyroid hormone for maintaining metabolic activity and energy. Both the overproduction of thyroid hormone, called hyperthyroidism, and the underproduction, hypothyroidism, can adversely affect the health of your skeleton. One of the most commonly ordered lab tests besides a comprehensive metabolic panel (CMP) and complete blood count (CBC) measures levels of thyroid-stimulating hormone (TSH), to assess the functioning of the thyroid gland. TSH is released by the pituitary gland in order to stimulate thyroid hormone production. When thyroid activity is lacking, TSH levels increase, and when thyroid hormone production is adequate, TSH levels decrease.

Both the overproduction of thyroid hormone as seen in Graves' disease and the overdosing of thyroid medication lead to thyrotoxicosis, a frequent cause of bone loss and heightened fracture risk. Thyrotoxicosis can be identified by very low levels of TSH. For years, doctors were only concerned about the overproduction of thyroid hormone as a contributor to bone loss in osteoporosis. Their interest in TSH levels was simply to rule out hyperthyroidism, and therefore they became concerned only if TSH levels were too low. But today we know that TSH is not just a sign of thyroid functioning; it actually affects the skeleton.

When there is too much TSH production, as seen in hypothyroidism, it will lead to bone loss. TSH doesn't just stimulate the thyroid gland, it increases the production of TNF, one of the most powerful pro-inflammatory cytokines and the one most responsible for increasing systemic inflammation. Even mild elevations of TSH, as seen in people with subclinical hypothyroidism, can negatively impact bone remodeling (Nagata et al. 2007).

EXERCISE 6.7: Signs and Symptoms of Excess Thyroid Hormone

In my patients with very low levels of TSH (indicating excessive thyroid hormone), I often find their bone density to be low.

In this exercise, if you highlight or check off three or more of the signs and symptoms of excess thyroid hormone (either from a hyper-functioning thyroid gland or too much thyroid medication), you may have abnormally low levels of TSH. Such excessive amounts of thyroid hormone within a person's system cause bone loss.

Signs and symptoms of excess thyroid hormone: Hyperactivity, tremor, weight loss, rapid, irregular heartbeat and bulging eyes.

EXERCISE 6.8: Signs and Symptoms of Low Thyroid Hormone

In my patients with very high levels of TSH (indicating low thyroid hormone), I often find their bone mineral density to be low. In exercise 6.8, if you highlight or check off three or more signs of low thyroid hormone (hypothyroidism), you may have abnormally high levels of TSH. Today, in certain cases, low production of thyroid hormone is also seen as causing bone loss.

Signs and symptoms of low thyroid hormone: Fatigue, weight gain (this is often absent in people with osteoporosis), cold hands and feet or sensitivity to cold, elevated cholesterol, difficulty concentrating, hair loss, dry skin, brittle nails, constipation, thinning of the eyebrows (especially the outer edges), depression, low body temperature, and low blood pressure.

Osteocalcin

You were introduced to the bone formation marker osteocalcin back in chapter 2. This important skeletal protein is produced by the osteoblasts during the bone formation phase of remodeling and is integral to bone mineralization. For that reason, osteocalcin can be a useful biomarker for assessing your response to treatment.

Osteocalcin doesn't just stimulate bone formation; it also acts as a hormone by playing a systemic role in the regulation of energy metabolism. A study at Columbia University (N. K. Lee et al. 2007) has shown that, in one sense, the skeleton is actually an endocrine organ whereby osteocalcin aids in the release of insulin from the pancreas. Therefore, the healthier your bones, the better your regulation of blood glucose will be and vice versa. Uncontrolled fluctuations of blood glucose in prediabetes or full-blown diabetes increase pro-inflammatory cytokines. This leads to systemic inflammation and bone loss.

Osteoporosis, which is characterized by poor production of osteocalcin and low osteoblastic activity, contributes to altered insulin control over blood glucose. Remember when I explained why it is so important to treat the underlying smoldering embers of osteoporosis and not just sprinkle on some bisphosphonate fire retardant? Systemic inflammation is the precursor to many diseases such as diabetes, not just osteoporosis. I hope you are now seeing the importance of this therapeutic approach.

Osteocalcin is not a hormone that can be prescribed. However, potassium, vitamin K, milk basic protein, berberine (an herbal alkaloid), rho-iso-alpha acids (RIAA), good nutrition to increase alkalinity, and supplemental support to reduce inflammation all help to increase osteocalcin production. Once produced, osteocalcin must be transformed by vitamin K into its activated form, carboxylated osteocalcin before it is able to promote bone formation. A laboratory test called undercarboxylated osteocalcin is available to determine if your vitamin K intake is sufficient for this activation of osteocalcin.

Serotonin and Melatonin

Made from the amino acid tryptophan, both serotonin and melatonin have roles in bone remodeling. Most people associate serotonin with the brain, where low levels reduce nerve activity, which leads to anxiety and depression. Selective serotonin reuptake inhibitors (SSRIs) are medications that block serotonin reuptake, thus improving nerve activity and stabilizing mood.

But brain serotonin is only 5 percent of what the body produces. The rest is formed in the gut, where it stimulates peristalsis, and, during the inflammatory response, increases vascular permeability. But overproduction of gut serotonin can cause problems. Overcolonization of undesirable microbes, or dysbiosis (Lord and Bralley 2008), as well as stress and irritable bowel conditions are prime contributors to overproduction. And chronic gut inflammation (e.g., inflammatory bowel and celiac disease) compromises serotonin reuptake mechanisms, thus allowing for its buildup (Costedio, Hyman, and Mawe 2007).

When gut levels of inflammation rise, whether from overproduction or a disruption of reuptake, the excess serotonin filters into the blood and heads for the skeleton. Scientists at Columbia University (Yadav et al. 2008) discovered that this serotonin inhibits osteoblastic bone formation. From there it's easy to see how excess production in the gut might limit tryptophan availability for the production of brain serotonin. No wonder that depression is considered a risk factor for osteoporosis. We've long known that using SSRIs to treat depression can lower bone density, but now we understand why—too much serotonin production in the gut inhibits osteoblast activity in bone. Maybe we should first look at reducing systemic inflammation and improving gastrointestinal health before reaching so quickly for those medications.

The hormone melatonin is formed in the brain's pineal gland, where it governs the sleep-wake cycle. Large amounts of melatonin are also produced within bone where, during stem cell differentiation, it guides the switch toward osteoblast cell formation and away from fat cell production (Sanchez-Hidalgo et al. 2007). For years, melatonin has been considered an antiaging hormone, but now we understand its role in preventing osteoporosis. Regular and restful sleep helps to normalize melatonin levels, and adequate melatonin limits excessive production of serotonin.

HORMONE THERAPY—IS IT RIGHT FOR YOU?

Deciding whether you should use estrogen (if you're a woman) or testosterone (if you're a man) for the treatment of your osteoporosis is simple. If you are considering hormone replacement therapy solely to improve your bone mineral density, the answer is "No, don't use it." There is no good evidence to indicate that HRT will reduce fractures in the long term, and hormone therapy is always accompanied by health risks.

On the other hand, if your osteoporosis is accompanied by symptoms of menopause, impotence, or other hormone-related conditions, then the question becomes more difficult to answer. Your doctor will be able to help you sift through all of the variables before you decide which option is best for you. Hormone replacement, when needed, can be of great benefit to improving your quality of life, and it may also positively affect the health of your skeleton. But keep in mind that although hormones may be the impulse behind life, their replacement in a body that is suffering from nutritional deficit, gastrointestinal ill health, or toxic overload will not produce a miracle cure.

TOXIC WATERS

If hormones are viewed as providing the energetic flow necessary for building strong bones, toxins can be seen as the source of their fouling. What was it that brought about the demise of health in Mr. Shea, from chapter 5? Were his poor muscle tone, stooped posture, depression, fatigue, and silently eroding bone caused simply by his sedentary lifestyle and poor nutrition? Could the mercury-laden amalgam fillings in his teeth have been involved in his catabolic wasting? And what about Ms. Lee? Certainly, she was putting a heavy toxic load into her body by smoking. Could a hidden toxin such as lead, a heavy metal well known to play havoc with hormones, have reduced her estrogen to a level that caused her to lose bone? In chapter 7, I'll cover several common toxins that can cause bone loss, the signs and symptoms that can signal their involvement, and what you can do about it if toxins are fouling your waters.

CHAPTER SEVEN

Environmental Toxins and Bone Loss

After the initial shock of being told I had severe osteoporosis, my first thought was "What is in my water that could do this to me?" For me to have osteoporosis something really weird had to have been going on. I was well aware of the Love Canal disaster. Was there something toxic in my own backyard? At Love Canal, the answer to the residents' mystifyingly high cancer rate had been in their water—maybe my answer would be found in my water supply too. The day after I got my diagnosis, I took a water sample from our 740-foot-deep well and took it to the local laboratory. I told the technician to run every test in the book.

OUR TOXIC WORLD

In retrospect, I wasn't totally wacky. We are all exposed daily to hundreds of toxins. If you're not being saturated by toxins from your own biological processes or those excreted by the bacteria and fungi within your GI tract, then you're being smothered by toxins in your external environment. It's not just urban areas that are polluted. No matter how far you travel, even to the far north where mercury-laden polar bears live, you cannot escape our toxic world.

For years, environmental pollutants have been known to cause cancer. Today we know that pollution also increases our overall level of inflammation and plays a major role in the development of chronic disease. A recent study (D. H. Lee et al. 2007) found that persistent organic pollutants are associated with type 2 diabetes, and that toxic metals, long known to interfere with vitamin D metabolism, contribute to bone loss. Recently, toxicants such as dioxins in pesticides, polycyclic aromatic hydrocarbons in cigarette smoke and automobile exhaust, and polychlorinated biphenyls in PVC piping and coolants have been linked to osteoporosis by interfering with osteoblast cell development (Ryan et al. 2007). Aluminum and the heavy metals lead, cadmium, and possibly mercury are the metals most frequently associated with osteoporosis.

Aluminum

Aluminum is in virtually everything. From cars and furniture to cookware, soda cans, food wraps, and even antacids, it is a daily part of everyone's life. Our awareness of aluminum's toxic effect on the skeleton stems from studies done with patients who required long-term dialysis for kidney disease. The fluids formerly used in dialysis contained high levels of aluminum and this caused extensive bone disease. Today, your greatest risk of aluminum-related bone loss would come from ingesting large amounts of aluminum-containing antacids.

For years, it was thought that because aluminum is efficiently excreted in the urine, it could reach toxic levels only in people with kidney disease. But we now know that aluminum, in a manner similar to lead, follows the absorption and deposition pathways of calcium. Therefore, the lower your calcium intake, the greater your aluminum absorption will be. When aluminum is absorbed, it goes directly into the bone, where it interferes with bone cell activity and the formation of the hydroxyapatite crystal (Malluche 2002). This leads to lower bone density and increased fracture risk. Aluminum-related bone loss can be seen even in people with normal kidney function.

Signs and symptoms of aluminum toxicity. These are the signs and symptoms of aluminum toxicity: osteoporosis or *osteomalacia* (a bone mineralization or softening disease commonly caused by a deficiency in vitamin D, known as rickets in children), hypersensitivity, irritability, short-term memory loss, anemia, Alzheimer's disease, and Parkinson's disease.

Sources of aluminum exposure. The primary source of potential toxicity is from antacids containing aluminum. Other sources include baking powder, aluminum-containing cookware, aluminum foil, processed foods, and contaminated water sources.

Laboratory testing for aluminum toxicity. These are the tests for aluminum toxicity: hair analysis, blood assay (only registers recent exposure and does not reflect the amount sequestered within bone), and bone biopsy (the only definitive test for diagnosing aluminum-related bone loss).

Therapy for aluminum toxicity. Chelation is a form of therapy for removing toxic metals. By infusing or orally administering special binding compounds, toxic metals can be captured and excreted from the body. Chelation therapy with desferrioxamine (DFO) or deferiprone (DMPH; Ferriprox) is recommended for aluminum toxicity (Blanuša et al. 2005).

Lead

Most of the attention to the ill effects of lead toxicity has focused on the neurological damage that it causes in children. Young, developing nervous systems are particularly vulnerable. But lead is also extremely toxic to adults even at low levels of exposure, and it places us at high risk for osteoporosis. In a study using data from the Third National Health and Nutrition Examination Survey, a definite association was found between blood lead levels and osteoporosis (Campbell and Auinger 2007). Lead disrupts enzyme function and reduces the osteoblasts' ability to form bone. It also reduces our ability to produce hormones such as testosterone and progesterone (Sierra and Tiffany-Castiglioni 1992).

Since lead was banned from paint in 1977 and phased out as an additive to gasoline in the 1980s, we tend to think it is no longer a health concern in the United States. But it is. Lead use continues in industry and in some sporting equipment, such as lead weights for fishing, and in making ammunition. It is still found in the plumbing systems and paint of older homes.

In addition to exposure through direct contact, there is another way that lead can be a risk to your health, and women are especially vulnerable. Let me explain. Lead is similar to calcium in that it is a bone-seeking element. When it is ingested or inhaled, lead competes with calcium for absorption and is deposited into bone. Lead accumulates in the body over time, and more than 90 percent of it is sequestered within the skeleton (Nash et al. 2004). For this reason, blood testing may not accurately reflect how much lead you have built up in your bones.

If you were exposed to high levels of lead as a child, it may still be sequestered in your bones, even if you are a premenopausal forty-five-year-old woman. It may be a hidden condition that blood tests would not reveal. At times of intense skeletal remodeling, such as during lactation and menopause, lead is released from bone into the bloodstream (Silbergeld et al. 1993). Because of this, when you enter menopause a blood test would then begin to show high levels of lead even with no additional exposure to the toxin.

As a result of this rise in blood lead level, you may experience a dramatic loss of BMD—a loss not due solely to the reduced estrogen of menopause, but due to lead's detrimental effects on the body's hormone production, enzymatic function, and bone cell activity. This increase in circulating lead has recently been shown (Khalil et al. 2008) to decrease hip BMD and to increase the risk for falls and fractures, even when blood levels are as low as 8 µg/dl, a concentration previously thought to be safe.

If you are presently within five to seven years after your menopause and you grew up in the 1940s, 1950s, or 1960s when lead was a more ubiquitous threat, you should ask your doctor to have you tested for lead toxicity, especially if you are experiencing brain fog, increased blood pressure, or a rapid loss of BMD. If this describes you, lead stored within your skeleton may be paying you a return visit. According to research performed at the University of Rochester Medical Center, such prior lead exposure, even decades ago, could place you at a higher risk for fracture (Carmouche et al. 2005).

Signs and symptoms of lead toxicity in the adult. These are some of the signs and symptoms of lead toxicity: irritability, abdominal pain, reduced attention span, memory loss, brain fog, metallic taste in mouth, pain, numbness, tingling in the extremities, fatigue, weakness, difficulty sleeping, loss of appetite, anemia, and a low sperm count.

Sources of lead exposure. These are some of the sources of lead exposure: water (from the plumbing systems of older houses), soil (around major highways and older homes), industry—battery and electronic manufacturing; cosmetics—this may be hard to believe, but certain products like lipstick can contain lead; remedies—herbal and calcium products from India and other parts of Asia; and hobbies—glazes, lead weights for fishing, and ammunition.

It's also good to remember that susceptibility to lead toxicity increases with low intake of calcium, zinc, iron, or magnesium.

Laboratory testing for lead toxicity. Hair and whole-blood analyses are the tests used for determining lead toxicity.

Therapy for lead toxicity. Oral or intravenous chelation therapy with ethylenediaminetetraacetic acid (EDTA) is the treatment for lead toxicity.

Cadmium

Cadmium is extremely toxic. Indeed, it is so toxic that Dr. Lars Järup (2002) of the Imperial College Faculty of Medicine in London states that disease, especially of the kidney and bone, is caused by cadmium exposure below the acceptable limits of 10 nmol (urine) set by the World Health Organization. In the Osteoporosis-Cadmium as a Risk Factor (OSCAR) study in the United Kingdom, it was determined that just 3 nmol of cadmium found in the urine indicated an exposure that was considered a risk for osteoporosis (Järup and Alfvén 2004). In a study from Poland, researchers determined that chronic low-level cadmium exposure, even at levels within the range of values seen in the general population, reduced bone density and increased fractures (Brzóska and Moniuszko-Jakoniuk 2004). Cadmium exposure is most common in proximity to fertilizers, industrial waste, automobile exhaust, jewelry making, and cigarette smoking.

Cadmium increases oxidative stress and pro-inflammatory cytokines (Dong et al. 1998). It also limits the osteoblast cell's ability to form bone collagen, disrupts vitamin D production in the kidneys, reduces progesterone levels, and stimulates the release of parathyroid hormone by reducing blood calcium levels.

Signs and symptoms of cadmium toxicity. Acute exposure to cadmium can cause symptoms of increased urination, chest pain, headache, and dizziness (Wittman and Hu 2002). But chronic low-level cadmium exposure may go unnoticed even though damage to the kidneys and bone is still taking place. The best method of determining whether cadmium is contributing to your bone loss is to assess your exposure and, if appropriate, be tested.

Sources of cadmium exposure. Foods such as vegetables and grains grown in cadmium-contaminated soil (whether contaminated by fertilizers or industrial waste) can expose you to toxic levels of cadmium. The following foods and environmental situations can also expose you to toxic levels: shellfish, canned foods, fish (especially from polluted rivers), cigarette smoke, automobile exhaust, and industries such as nickel-cadmium battery manufacturing. Iron-deficient anemia puts you at a higher risk, as does zinc deficiency.

Laboratory testing for cadmium toxicity. The tests for cadmium toxicity are hair analysis, urine, and blood (for recent exposure only).

Therapy for cadmium toxicity. Oral or intravenous chelation therapy for the treatment of cadmium toxicity includes EDTA, dimercaptosuccinic acid (DMSA), and N-acetyl cysteine (Blanuša et al. 2005).

Mercury

If you ever want to start a heated discussion, just mention mercury toxicity to a group of medical professionals. No one doubts mercury's toxicity, but exactly to what extent this heavy metal influences disease is a hotly debated topic. Mercury exposure is known to damage the kidneys, liver, nervous tissue, and the brain. It has been implicated in autoimmune disease, cardiovascular disease, and neurodegenerative diseases such as Alzheimer's, Parkinson's, multiple sclerosis, and autism.

Mercury's involvement as a causative agent in osteoporosis has not been established. But interestingly, there are several mechanisms whereby mercury toxicity may have the potential to cause harm by disrupting the delicately coupled system of bone remodeling. Mercury increases oxidative stress (it increases lipid peroxides), depletes antioxidants, replaces zinc in critical enzymes thereby diminishing their actions, and may reduce the effectiveness of progesterone and other hormones (Quig 1998). Does mercury toxicity contribute to bone loss? Only future research will be able to fully delineate its effects on the skeleton.

Signs and symptoms of mercury toxicity. These are the signs and symptoms of mercury toxicity: chronic fatigue, depression, brain fog, poor memory, tingling or numbness in the extremities, and chronic yeast infections.

Sources of mercury exposure. These are the sources of mercury exposure: fish (both fresh water and saltwater), dental amalgam fillings, and thimerosal (a preservative in vaccines).

Laboratory testing for mercury toxicity. Tests for mercury toxicity include hair analysis and a provoked urine test using DMSA (2, 3-dimercaptosuccinic acid). Note: because mercury is sequestered within the body's soft tissues, an agent such as DMSA is needed to provoke (mobilize) it and bring it into the blood and urine where it can be measured. Urinary porphyrins can also be measured. *Porphyrins* are the oxidized products of various compounds made up of organic chemical and metal molecules. Excreted from the body, they can be used as biomarkers to assess the effects of toxic metals. Not used to identify specific toxins, they can be used to verify the presence of toxic metals within someone with clinical symptoms suspected to be toxin related.

Therapy for mercury toxicity. Methods for dealing with mercury toxicity include removing the source of mercury (e.g., amalgam fillings) and then chelation therapy with DMSA or dimercaptopropanesolfunate (DMPS). Overall nutritional support can enhance the excretion of mercury through the feces. Specific oral supplemements, such as selenium (Fitzgerald, Nelson-Dooley, and Lord 2008), N-acetyl cysteine, alphalipoic acid, and glutathione (Patrick 2002) can be helpful in chelating mercury and reducing its damaging effects.

Iron

Any metal taken in excess, even iron, is toxic to the body. Iron isn't considered an environmental pollutant, but it must be mentioned because it has the potential to contribute to your bone loss. It's hard to imagine, but the iron supplement your mother insisted on as a safeguard against anemia actually can harm you if taken in excess. Iron accumulation leads to heart and liver disease and possibly even to cancer (Stevens et al. 1988). As we age, our oxidative stress levels increase and excessive iron intake increases the production of free radicals, which create more oxidative damage. In a study performed on animals at the University of Utah School of Medicine, researchers concluded that iron overload suppresses bone formation and stimulates bone resorption (Liu et al. 2008). The important lesson to take from this study is that if you're postmenopausal and taking iron supplements, make sure that your blood tests indicate a need for iron.

DON'T GET OVERWHELMED!

It's easy to get worried because so many different toxins can cause osteoporosis. Relax; you are still gathering the information you'll need to combat your bone loss. Environmental toxins are one tiny piece of a much larger puzzle. Most people will have no need to be tested, but you should be aware of the possibility. If you think you have been exposed to an environmental toxin, talk with your doctor about appropriate testing. A urine toxic element test can easily help identify and monitor toxic levels of lead, cadmium, aluminum, and mercury. Several of the specialty labs listed in the Resources section can perform this type of testing. The most important action you can take is to avoid toxins. Here are some suggestions that will help you to see the big picture of metal toxicity as it pertains to your bone health:

- *Aluminum:* If you take antacids with high levels of aluminum, switch to a brand with less, then work with your doctor to eliminate the causes of your stomach upset (for example, food allergies or the need for digestive aids). Never cook with aluminum pots or pans.

- *Lead:* If you've had chronic exposure to lead (even as a child), have your blood tested.

- *Cadmium:* If you smoke, quit.

- *Mercury:* If your diet has included high amounts of fish or you have a mouthful of amalgam fillings, consider a DMSA provoked urine test to assess the level of mercury in your body.

- *Iron:* If you are postmenopausal, most likely you won't want to be taking any extra iron. Check to make sure that the multivitamin you use does not include iron. If you think you may be deficient in iron, check with your doctor so that he or she can order a lab test to assess your need.

CHAPTER EIGHT

Bone-Specific Pharmaceuticals for Reducing Fracture Risk

Every wilderness trek has its potential for disaster. But if you've prepared properly and you assess each dangerous situation individually, in all probability you will emerge unscathed and stronger both physically and emotionally. Survival is about being smart and doing what is necessary at that particular moment for that particular problem with your particular ability. Survival is not about doing what others did before you. Practicing patience and avoiding panic will always help you make the right decisions. But deciding if and when to use drug therapy to treat bone loss can be plagued with difficult questions like these:

- Can hormone therapy help reduce your risk for fracture or will it just increase the risk for breast cancer and heart disease?

- Is it okay to start taking a bisphosphonate at the age of fifty when it may lead to brittle bones when you're in your seventies?

- Does your particular T score really place you at risk for a fracture, or is there wiggle room before you have to start taking a medication?

- What exactly is osteonecrosis of the jaw and what is your risk of getting it if you take a bisphosphonate?

- Should you consider using parathyroid hormone therapy when it potentially could stimulate cancer growth?

If you have osteoporosis and are considering the use of a medication, you already may be asking some of these questions. Unfortunately, there are no blanket answers because every one of you is unique. The best you can do is combine your newfound knowledge of bone biology with the information in this chapter and then sit down with your doctor to discuss your options. He or she will be your best guide for determining your optimal course of action. The rest of this chapter explains the pros and cons of using the medications currently available to treat bone loss.

CURRENT RECOMMENDATIONS FOR DRUG THERAPY INTERVENTION

In 2007, the World Health Organization (WHO) developed a fracture risk assessment tool (FRAX) to help predict fractures in men and women (Kanis et al. 2008). This new algorithm does not rely on BMD T scores. Instead, the WHO assessment looked at clinical risk factors such as body mass index (BMI), prior history of fracture, parental history of hip fracture, medications, preexisting diseases, and lifestyle factors in order to assess a person's ten-year fracture risk. Based on this new tool, the National Osteoporosis Foundation (NOF) has recommended the following guidelines to help clinicians identify those individuals who need drug therapy. These guidelines address postmenopausal women and men age fifty and older (National Osteoporosis Foundation 2008):

- Individuals with a hip or vertebral fracture

- Individuals who have experienced any other fractures and who have a T score between -1.0 and -2.5

- Individuals with a T score of -2.5 or lower at the hip or spine after they have been evaluated for secondary causes

- Individuals with a T score between -1.0 and -2.5 at the hip or spine with secondary factors associated with high fracture risk

- Individuals with a T score between -1.0 and -2.5 at the hip or spine and a ten-year probability of 3 percent or greater for a hip fracture, or a ten-year probability of any major osteoporosis-related fracture of 20 percent or greater based on the WHO algorithm

The NOF emphasizes that these guidelines are to be used only as a basic reference and that actual treatment recommendations should be tailored to the individual patient's needs.

The pharmaceutical industry would like you to begin using their drugs sooner rather than later. In one of those all-too-common uncomfortable alignments of drug companies with medical policy makers, the 1994 WHO study group that defined osteoporosis as having a T score of -2.5 was funded by several major drug companies (World Health Organization 1994). But we know that determining fracture risk on the basis of T scores is not accurate. So why should you rely on your T score as the only marker to determine the use of medications? In deciding when and if to use drug therapy, it is your particular situation that must be assessed—not just your T score.

There is no doubt that osteoporosis-specific medications help reduce fracture risk—at least in the short term. Medications can be powerful and extremely helpful but should be used only when necessary. In one study (Schousboe et al. 2005), bisphosphonates were not shown to be cost-effective for treating postmenopausal women with femoral neck T scores of -2.5 or better and no history of fracture. Today, concern is growing that if bisphosphonates are taken for too many years, a buildup of microfractures may cause the skeleton to become brittle. There is a similar concern in that these drugs may lead to osteonecrosis of the jaw (Ruggiero et al. 2004).

When considering the use of medications for your low BMD, proceed with caution. Talk to your doctor about their benefits and risks, and make your decision based on the course of action that best suits your situation. You might benefit most by using a bisphosphonate for three years and then taking a drug holiday. Or you might use teriparatide for one year and then begin a bisphosphonate. The options vary. What matters is that you should use medications wisely and only when needed. Think of them as emergency provisions—not as a steady diet.

CURRENTLY APPROVED DRUG THERAPIES FOR OSTEOPOROSIS

The Food and Drug Administration (FDA) has approved quite a few prescription medicines to prevent and treat postmenopausal osteoporosis and osteoporosis in men. But currently there are no FDA-approved therapies for premenopausal osteoporosis. None. Here is a list of medications currently available.

Bisphosphonates: alendronate (Fosamax); risedronate (Actonel); ibandronate (Boniva)—approved only for postmenopausal women; zoledronate (Reclast)—a once-a-year intravenous infusion for postmenopausal women.

Selective estrogen receptor modulators (SERMS): raloxifene (Evista)— approved only for women.

Calcitonin: calcitonin-salmon (Calcimar, Fortical [nasal spray] and Miacalcin [nasal spray or injection]).

Parathyroid hormone: teriparatide (Forteo)

Hormone replacement (women): conjugated equine estrogens (Climera, Estrace, Estraderm, Ogen, Ortho-Est, Premarin, Vivelle); conjugated equine estrogens plus progestin (Activella, Femhrt, Premphase, Prempro); bioidentical estrogen; progestin; bioidentical progesterone.

Strontium: strontium ranelate (Protelos)—developed in France, not available in the United States; strontium gluconate, strontium carbonate, strontium lactate, and strontium chloride—all available in nonprescription supplement form.

Hormone replacement (men): testosterone (Testoderm; Androderm) —recommended only for osteoporosis related to extremely low testosterone production.

BISPHOSPHONATES

Bone health is naturally maintained in your body by a balanced remodeling system. Osteoblasts must form enough bone to replace what was resorbed by the osteoclasts. Keeping this system in balance is the only way that bone health can be maintained. In an attempt to correct the imbalance that leads to bone loss, the pharmaceutical industry has concentrated on developing drugs that reduce overly aggressive osteoclastic activity. The result has been the development of several generations of bisphosphonates with increasing potency. Although effective in boosting BMD, if you listen to the many commercials on TV, you might think bisphosphonate medications are also the key to eternal youth. The truth is that bisphosphonates are only *antiresorptive* agents. They prevent osteoclasts from resorbing bone. That's all they do. They don't provide energy or strength, and they don't reduce inflammation or renew your vitality. But they can get you out of a bind.

How Do Bisphosphonates Work?

Bisphosphonates are chemical cousins of the inorganic pyrophosphates that have been used for years to soften water and remove the buildup of mineral scaling in pipes. Just as pyrophosphates bind to minerals in water to make it "soft," bisphosphonates bind to the calcium in the hydroxyapatite crystal of bone. It's here that bisphosphonates can curtail excessive osteoclast activity. Osteoclasts are quite a lot like coyotes. They scavenge old and worn-out bone so that new, stronger bone can be made. Coyotes scavenge dead or dying animals and are integral to the ecology of a forest. When farmers want to kill off the local coyotes, they lace meat with poisons. When doctors want to kill off osteoclasts, they lace your bones with bisphosphonates. These medications, when absorbed by the osteoclasts, repress their activity and eventually destroy them. With fewer osteoclasts, bone resorption is limited and fracture risk is diminished.

What Are the Side Effects of Bisphosphonate Use?

As with any medication, there can be minor and major side effects. The minor side effects commonly experienced with oral bisphosphonates are stomach pain, muscle pain, bone and joint pain, diarrhea, gas, indigestion, and nausea. More serious side effects can include esophagitis (inflammation of the throat) and even ulcerations of the stomach, which are not uncommon. In January 2008, the FDA released an alert concerning bisphosphonate use that warned of the possibility of severe and sometimes incapacitating and long-lasting bone, joint, or muscle pain. Also, the agency is currently investigating concerns that these medications may contribute to atrial fibrillation, a disorder of the heart's rhythms.

Ironically, bisphosphonates have been associated with contributing to a higher fracture rate in a specific situation: because oral bisphosphonates often cause GERD-like stomach and throat pain, doctors may prescribe proton pump inhibitors (PPIs) with the bisphosphonate to control side effects. A recent study (de Vries et al. 2008) determined that the combined use of bisphosphonates and PPIs increased fractures when compared to using bisphosphonates alone.

Intravenous bisphosphonates can cause transient fever, muscle pain, eye inflammation, optic neuritis, and blood clots at the injection site. The most alarming complication from either oral or intravenous bisphosphonates, however, is osteonecrosis of the jaw.

OSTEONECROSIS OF THE JAW

Osteonecrosis means "death of bone tissue." In osteonecrosis of the jaw (ONJ), the bones holding your teeth lose their ability to remodel because of what appears to be an oversuppression of osteoclastic activity by bisphosphonate medications. The jawbone becomes exposed and cannot heal. The areas of exposed bone are resistant to medical treatment and often become infected, leading to chronic, intractable pain and disfigurement. Discontinuing the bisphosphonate does nothing to improve a patient's response to therapy. Treatment in such cases of ONJ remains supportive at best.

Although ONJ is most commonly seen in cancer patients receiving intravenous bisphosphonates (one to ten cases per 100 patients), it is also seen in those using oral bisphosphonates. We don't know the exact risk for contracting ONJ with oral bisphosphonate use, but it does appear to be exceedingly low. Dr. John Bilezikian, professor of medicine and pharmacology at Columbia University, estimates the incidence to be somewhere between 1 in 100,000 and 1 in 250,000 patient-treatment years (Lewiecki et al. 2008).

There are measures that may help to prevent bisphosphonate-associated ONJ. If you are considering using a bisphosphonate, it's essential to maintain good oral hygiene. This encourages a neutral pH and a healthy bacteria population in your oral cavity, which better allows tissues to repair and maintain their structural integrity. Also, while you use a bisphosphonate, it would be a good idea to have your doctor monitor your bone turnover markers. Although a recent study (Farooki, Fornnier, and Estilo 2008) did not see consistently low resorption markers in cancer patients who developed ONJ after treatment with intravenous bisphosphonates, this method to identify those at risk for ONJ while taking an oral bisphosphonate for osteoporosis treatment is the best tool we have at the present time. If you are taking a bisphosphonate and a resorption marker indicates that your bone remodeling is being oversuppressed, your doctor may suggest a drug holiday.

Long-Term Bisphosphonate Use

Bisphosphonates interrupt the tightly coupled choreography of bone cells during remodeling. The reduction in bone turnover leads to skeletal aging, and there are concerns that long-term use (more than three years) may lead to increased microfractures and brittle bones. If people start taking bisphosphonates when they are thirty, forty, or even fifty years old, by the time they reach their seventies it would be difficult to describe their skeleton as healthy.

Using Bisphosphonates to Get You Out of a Bind

I'm glad I didn't start taking bisphosphonates at the age of forty-five to the exclusion of a nutrition program. But I did take a bisphosphonate for a short time (five months). I was breaking bones so often that I had to do something quickly. All it took was for me to simply lean against a fence or play an easy game of soccer with my son, and I would break another rib. I had to apply emergency intervention to stop the crumbling of my bones.

Bisphosphonates can be extremely useful medications and should be used when appropriate. Creating change with nutrition has its limits. Changing your physiology takes time. Improving bone health through nutrition can be slow, and for some, genetics or advancing age may prove insurmountable. In addition, adverse cellular changes within a stressed physiology can become permanent. For example, the development of RANKL-expressing memory cells (special immune cells) within the bone marrow may perpetuate bone loss even with the best in nutritional therapy. So don't be afraid to use a bisphosphonate to pull yourself out of danger if need be. Just be on the lookout for adverse symptoms. Sensible bisphosphonate therapy can offer you benefits that far outweigh the risks, including the risk of contracting ONJ.

■ *Ms. Lee*

Ms. Lee, a svelte sixty-eight-year-old clothing store owner, came into my office with a history of diarrhea, bloating, and abdominal pain following a vacation in Mexico. A year before her trip to Mexico, a DXA exam had indicated that Ms. Lee's BMD was very low (T scores: spine -3.1 and hips -2.0). Now, after six months of abdominal pain and two courses of medi-

cations to treat a parasitic infection, a second DXA exam, less than two years after the first, revealed that her bone density had plummeted. Her spine T score was now -3.8 and her hips were -2.5. Obviously, Ms. Lee was not absorbing nutrients, and her bone resorption biomarker, NTX, was extremely high at 198 nmol. Indeed, she was not only unable to build bone, she was losing bone rapidly.

Alarmed, with good reason, Ms. Lee's primary care doctor prescribed alendronate to stop osteoclasts from resorbing excessive amounts of her bone. But to prescribe only a bisphosphonate and not address the cause of her rapid bone loss would be short-sighted. Alendronate would reduce Ms. Lee's immediate danger of fracturing (as indicated by her low T scores as well as her elevated NTX) but nutritional support would bring her bones, as well as her whole body, to an improved state of health.

After pinpointing her dysbiosis as a prime source of her systemic inflammation, we were able to relieve her gastrointestinal distress and reduce her acutely elevated markers of inflammation and oxidative stress. We used the 4R program and supported her body with vitamins, minerals, amino acids, and essential fatty acids. After Ms. Lee had been on this therapeutic regime for several months I repeated her NTX test. This time it showed a dramatic reduction—a fall from a disturbing 198 nmol to a more normal 48 nmol—indicating less inflammation and less bone loss. This definitely showed that Ms. Lee was getting healthier.

With her systemic inflammation reduced and a well-balanced diet and supplement program in place, we would continually monitor Ms. Lee's progress over the next several years. If her biomarkers continued to improve and she suffered no fractures, hopefully, we would be able to reduce or even eliminate her prescription for alendronate.

SELECTIVE ESTROGEN RECEPTOR MODULATORS

SERMs (selective estrogen receptor modulators) act similarly to estrogen while avoiding some of the adverse reactions that often accompany estrogen therapy. The only FDA-approved SERM to prevent and treat osteoporosis is raloxifene (Evista). It is an option for women unable to tolerate bisphosphonates, or those who prefer to avoid hormone therapy, or for whom estrogen therapy is contraindicated. Raloxifene is estrogenic in that it helps maintain bone density and lowers cholesterol, but it is antiestrogenic on breast and uterine tissue. Several studies have shown it to reduce the incidence of estrogen receptor-positive breast cancer (Cummings et al. 1999; Martino et al. 2004). Although raloxifene does increase BMD and reduce spinal fractures, it has not been shown to reduce hip, forearm, or other fractures.

Raloxifene therapy is sometimes accompanied by hot flashes, leg cramps, flu-like symptoms, swelling, and venous thromboembolism (blood clots).

CALCITONIN

Calcitonin is a hormone secreted by the thyroid gland for the purpose of directing blood calcium into bone. Salmon calcitonin, primarily administered as a nasal spray, was one of the first medications developed specifically to treat osteoporosis. It can be prescribed to osteoporotic men who have normal testosterone levels and to women who are five years beyond menopause and unable to take bisphosphonates. It reduces bone resorption by limiting osteoclastic activity. Therefore, it lowers calcium levels in the blood and keeps the calcium in the skeleton.

Nasal calcitonin has been shown to reduce vertebral fractures and appears to be of particular benefit to elderly women with osteoporosis, although its ability to reduce nonvertebral fractures has not been demonstrated (Chesnut et al. 2008). In the largest study to date on the effectiveness of nasal calcitonin, the Prevent Recurrence of Osteoporotic Fractures (PROOF) trial failed to demonstrate conclusively that calcitonin reduced fractures (Chesnut et al. 2000).

In a more recent study, researchers from the University of Washington Medical Center tested the effects of nasal spray salmon calcitonin over a two-year period. They determined that there was a significant improvement in trabecular microarchitecture in bones of the hip and forearm and a 22.5 percent reduction in bone resorption markers, even though there was no significant increase in BMD compared to the control group (Chesnut et al. 2005).

Calcitonin therapy is a good option to consider, especially if you can't tolerate bisphosphonate therapy or are uncomfortable with the risk of developing bisphosphonate-induced ONJ. Calcitonin seems to be very safe. It's an attractive therapeutic option if you are experiencing pain from an osteoporosis-related fracture. Several studies have demonstrated that it can reduce back pain caused by osteoporosis-related compression fractures (Lyritis et al. 1991).

PARATHYROID HORMONE

Teriparatide (Forteo) is a genetically manufactured portion of the parathyroid hormone molecule. Unlike bisphosphonates, which simply prevent osteoclasts from resorbing bone, teriparatide is considered an anabolic medication because it actually builds bone tissue. It is only for those who have both severe osteoporosis (T score less than -3.0) and a high risk for fracture. The FDA has placed a "black box" warning on teriparatide stating that it carries a significant risk of serious adverse effects. For this reason, its use for an individual has been restricted to a maximum of two years.

Teriparatide is currently taken as a self-administered daily injection. If parathyroid hormone were secreted continuously into your body, it would cause your bones to break down. But a limited, daily injection actually builds bone. It really works. Teriparatide has been shown to significantly increase bone mineral density in the spine and hip, and to dramatically reduce both spinal and nonspinal fractures.

If you are contemplating teriparatide use, you might consider monitoring its effectiveness. A few people do not respond to teriparatide at all. Others may respond initially with rapid bone formation that then dwindles after six months to a year. You don't want to keep treating yourself with this medication if it isn't helping. Fortunately, it's possible to monitor teriparatide's efficacy through the bone formation marker P1NP.

If P1NP levels suddenly fall, this indicates that your body is no longer responding anabolically. It is possible then (with your physician's guidance) to pulse your treatment to enhance the drug's benefit. Allow me to explain:

If your initial response to teriparatide was positive (indicated by a rise in P1NP), but its effectiveness has dwindled (indicated by a P1NP reduction), then taking a break for six months to a year will give your body a rest from the rigors of bone production. During this interval, your doctor will prescribe a bisphosphonate to prevent the rapid loss of bone density that usually occurs when teriparatide is stopped (this is called sequential drug therapy). Teriparatide can be tough on the body. It forces it to do something (build bone) it finds difficult (otherwise you wouldn't have osteoporosis). Some individuals' bodies just scream, "No more!" to teriparatide's "request" to build bone. Not taking it for an extended period (while making sure to take a bisphosphonate), and then reinstating teriparatide injections may be all you need to regain its anabolic effects. With treatment limited to two years, it's essential to use this drug to its greatest advantage.

HORMONE REPLACEMENT THERAPY FOR WOMEN

Currently, estrogen and hormone replacement therapy has been discouraged for any reason other than the short-term alleviation of menopausal symptoms. This is due to the disturbing results from the Women's Health Initiative study, which determined that the risks of heart disease, stroke, clotting, and breast cancer from using HRT outweighed its benefits. Estrogen and other hormone replacement therapy for postmenopausal osteoporosis should be used only in the lowest effective doses for the shortest time possible.

If you are experiencing severe postmenopausal symptoms and have osteoporosis, hormone replacement therapy with bioidentical hormones may be a sensible therapeutic option. If you have not had a hysterectomy, progesterone should be included in your monthly cycle of estrogen replacement to help reduce your risk of endometrial cancer. And, of course, even with bioidentical hormones, you should still use the lowest effective dose for the shortest duration.

HORMONE REPLACEMENT THERAPY FOR MEN

Low estrogen levels in women are clearly related to increased fracture risk, but the effects of low testosterone on bone in both sexes are less defined. As men age, their blood levels of pro-inflammatory cytokines rise and their testosterone levels fall. This indicates that low testosterone has a role in the inflammation symptoms seen with aging and with bone loss. But the relationship of low testosterone to increased fracture risk hasn't yet been clearly delineated. Testosterone replacement for men who have osteoporosis is therefore recommended only when blood levels fall below 300 ng/dl or when symptoms clearly indicate the need for supplementation.

STRONTIUM

A study of 1,649 postmenopausal women (Meunier et al. 2004) concluded that 2 grams per day of oral strontium ranelate (Protelos) reduced fracture risk by 50 percent. Strontium ranelate is not available in the United States; however, one study (Genuis and Schwalfenberg 2007) showed that strontium gluconate, strontium carbonate, strontium lactate, and strontium chlorate may also promote a positive effect on bone. Numerous animal studies have demonstrated positive changes to bone structure using these forms of strontium, but to date there have been no large-scale human studies (Marie et al. 1985; Shahnazari et al. 2006). Strontium ranelate decreases bone resorption and stimulates new bone formation. This combination of antiresorptive and anabolic actions creates stronger and more fracture-resistant bone. So high levels of strontium may be an appropriate addition to your specific strategic nutrition-based therapeutic regime.

OSTEOPOROSIS DRUGS ON THE HORIZON

Currently, several new drugs for the prevention and treatment of osteoporosis are either in late-stage clinical trials or under review for FDA approval. These include an antiresorptive drug called denosumab, and three next-generation SERMs.

Denosumab is a manufactured human antibody against RANKL. This drug can inhibit bone resorption not by disabling osteoclasts as bisphosphonates do, but by prohibiting their actual development. (You learned in chapter 4 that RANKL increases bone loss by stimulating osteoclast cell maturation.) The problem with removing RANKL is that this cytokine is involved in both bone remodeling and white blood cell activation. Its absence may increase the incidence of infection and tumor growth. If the FDA becomes convinced of denosumab's efficacy and safety, it will likely grant approval in 2009.

Pharmaceutical companies are always searching for the perfect SERM—one that would reduce the incidence of hip fractures, breast cancer, cardiovascular disease, and dementia without causing endometrial cancer, hot flashes, or venous thromboembolisms. The three new SERMs on the horizon are lasofoxifene (Fablyn), bazedoxifene (Viviant), and arzoxifene. Although these estrogenic compounds may be an improvement over raloxifene (Evista), none has yet shown a reduction in hip fractures, and all have pending safety concerns.

ANABOLIC PHYSIOLOGY: RENEWING SKELETAL HEALTH

One of my deepest frustrations as a doctor is seeing people lulled into the misconception that a medication will make them healthy. Osteoporosis medications are to be used for the purpose of reducing fracture risk. They do not supply you with nutrients, nor do they reduce your oxidative stress. They don't make you anabolic, and they sure don't make you healthy. In the next chapter I'll summarize the most important steps for you to take to improve the health of your bones. The process actually comes down to one thing only—nurturing an anabolic physiology. That is the key to renewing skeletal health.

CHAPTER NINE

How to Create an Anabolic Body

No matter who you are, if you walk deeply into the forest enough times, you're going to get lost. I certainly have—several times. Dark, twisting ravines, steeply sloped hillsides, and impenetrable tangles can be disorienting. That's the bad news. The good news is that if you persist, if you meet each obstacle as only an exaggerated distortion in the context of the whole forest, then your thoughts will remain centered and you'll successfully find your way.

To reduce my fracture risk I had to do more than just make my bones heavier with calcium. I had to reduce the chronic systemic inflammation in my body that was putting me at risk for other chronic degenerative disease; I had to make my body more alkaline, less wasteful, and more receptive to the resources provided by food and supplements; and I had to keep my tissues supple and muscles strong so that as I age, I will have less risk of falling. I needed to first uncover and then rectify the causes of the catabolic process that permeated my entire unhealthy body. I found no magic bullets to fix my osteoporosis. Magic bullets in this arena are rare.

Although I advocate the use of lifestyle and dietary changes along with nutritional supplementation as the first choice for improving your skeletal and overall health, medications can help to reduce your fracture risk. But please use them wisely. In the long run they won't fix your body's intricately troubled, catabolic web, which took years of physiological imbalance to weave. The only magic I've ever discovered came with persistence and openness to all forms of healing. But that's not magic, is it? Isn't that just being pragmatic?

IT'S ALL ABOUT BECOMING ANABOLIC

By now you realize that calcium and vitamin D, although integral to your skeletal health, may do you little good if your body is catabolic and in a constant state of destruction. Eliminating chronic, low-level metabolic acidosis, excess oxidative stress, systemic inflammation, and gastrointestinal dysfunction are far more useful for healing purposes than overloading your body with calcium. Your major objective, instead of simply swallowing a few key nutrients, should now be to build up your whole body—to become anabolic.

Find a Health Care Provider Who Will Work with You

Finding a compatible health care provider may take some effort, but it's crucial. The health care provider you choose to help you with your skeletal health should be knowledgeable about nutrition and laboratory testing and should be willing to take the time necessary to manage your case. Remember that osteoporosis is a chronic condition and requires a long-term, thorough, and vigilant approach.

Eat Healthy Food and Maintain a Positive, Constructive Attitude

Your goal is to improve the health of your entire body. If you succeed with your soft tissues, your bones will follow suit. It doesn't matter if you're fifty or eighty years old, if you want your body to respond, you need to care for it 24/7. Always remember that you want to make yourself stronger, more coordinated, and more capable. To do that, you must avoid harmful lifestyle activities and concentrate on foods that are healthy for you.

The foods you eat are your foundation for recovery. Consume predominately fruits and vegetables with lots of fiber. Be diligent about limiting your intake of refined sugars and other bone-robbing foods. Cook with healthy oils like olive and organic virgin coconut oil. Make sure you eat good-quality protein and that you include some protein with every meal. Eggs, poultry, fish, nuts, legumes, and whey or hemp powder are your best sources.

Go easy on red meat. If your body is catabolic, a daily consumption of 1.2 to 1.5 grams of quality lean protein per kilogram of your body weight will help you to become anabolic. Since a kilogram is equal to 2.2 pounds, if you weigh 125 pounds, that's between 70 and 85 grams of protein a day. If you are like me and weigh in at about 150 pounds, your protein requirement would be between 80 and 100 grams a day. Protein will increase the level of IGF-1 hormone in your blood, help you gain muscle tissue and strength, and provide you with the amino acids necessary for bone collagen formation. Caution: If you suffer from kidney disease, consult your doctor before increasing your protein intake.

Goals are great motivators. Set a mental or physical challenge for yourself—something to stretch your abilities, something to reach for. Train for a walkathon, road race, or triathlon; write a story or a journal article; or take up a new activity.

Use Nutritional Supplements to Boost Skeletal Health

Refer frequently to the list of key bone nutrients in the appendix. Doing that will help you stay aware of deficiency signs and symptoms, pertinent laboratory biomarkers, and dietary sources of nutrients and their recommended daily intakes. Even if your diet is impeccable, the fact that you have bone loss puts you into the special needs category. Now your body requires more than what you can get from diet alone. You should take the following as minimal supplementation:

- Multivitamin-mineral

- Calcium (1,000 to 1,200 mg/day)

- Magnesium (500 to 600 mg/day)

- Vitamin D_3 (1,000 to 2,000 IU/day)

- Vitamin K (1 mg/day or more)

- Antioxidant supplement (a broad-spectrum product such as vitamins C and E, selenium, N-acetyl cysteine, leucine, alpha-lipoic acid, and curcumin)

- Fish oil (2 to 3 gm/day); flaxseed meal (2 to 4 tablespoons/day)

- Probiotics (3 to 20 billion viable cells/day)

HOW TO FIND QUALITY NUTRITIONAL SUPPLEMENTS

Professional lines of nutritional and herbal supplements are of better quality than those sold in retail or health food stores. Ask your doctor if he or she has access to professional-quality supplements; if not, refer to the Resources section. A good company will gladly supply you with a certificate of analysis on their products. This certificate ensures that their products contain exactly what is printed on the label and only what is on the label, and that the products are free of contaminants and heavy metals. The company should be able to send you this certificate by e-mail within twenty-four hours. If not, find a different company. In addition to a certificate of analysis, the very best companies can provide you with information regarding their own quality control testing. You might pay a little more for their products, but they're worth it.

Start Your Therapeutic Targets Chart

If you haven't already started your therapeutic targets chart (described in exercises 2.1 and 4.1), do it now. This will help you understand where you are and where you're going in the management of your bone loss. Chart your signs and symptoms and correlate them to nutritional deficiencies or physiological dysfunction. Ask your doctor to help you. When your doctor orders laboratory tests, he or she will probably use one of the larger companies such as LabCorp or Quest for the basic core biomarkers. For some of the specialty tests, such as stool analysis, IgG allergy testing, and 8OH2dG, your doctor will need to seek the services of a laboratory that performs functional testing. In the Resources section, I've listed several reputable companies that I use for these purposes.

Has Your Doctor Ordered the Basic Core of Laboratory Tests?

Talk with your doctor about obtaining the basic core of laboratory tests for evaluating low bone density. Of course, he or she may want to do more extensive testing if it is needed. The basic core tests, discussed in chapter 2, consists of the following tests:

- Comprehensive metabolic panel (CMP).

- Complete blood count (CBC).

- Vitamin D [25(OH)D].

- Urine pH (morning).

- Urine calcium (either a calcium to creatinine ratio or a twenty-four-hour urine calcium test).

- Celiac profile (consisting of anti-tissue transglutaminase and antigliadin antibodies).

- Some form of bone resorption biomarker (NTX, CTX, or DPD).

Do a Monthly Check of Your Acid-Alkaline Balance

A diet too high in protein from cheese, meat, and grain products will lead to chronic low-level metabolic acidosis and ensuing bone loss. Study your food intake over a four-day period. Write down everything you eat. If your diet is too high in protein or especially heavy in grains and lacking in fruits and vegetables, make some changes. Increase your intake of high-potassium alkaline foods like broccoli, prunes, bok choy, kale, and squash.

Get into the habit of checking your first morning urine. This should be done every month for three to four days in a row. You're aiming for an average pH of 6.6 to 7.5. If your pH is consistently below 6.0 even with an improved diet, try supplementing for a month or two with potassium citrate or potassium bicarbonate. When your urine pH stabilizes above 6.6, discontinue the potassium supplements but continue eating lots of fruits and vegetables.

Ensure Your Gastrointestinal Health

Listen to your body. Are there signs and symptoms of poor gut health? Check with your doctor if you have *any* concerns. He or she will be able to order tests such as a stool analysis or a screening for food allergies. If you have osteoporosis, you should be tested for gluten sensitivity even if you have no gastrointestinal signs or symptoms. For gut health, the following points are the most important:

- Supplement each meal with hydrochloric acid or digestive enzymes, if needed.

- If your signs and symptoms indicate a need, check for food sensitivities or allergies. You can use either an elimination diet or food allergy testing (IgE and IgG testing) to rule out food allergies. If you have any indication that you may be sensitive to gluten, do not pass Go, do not collect $200; simply eliminate gluten from your diet immediately.

- If you're harboring abnormal gut microbes, you may require stool analysis testing. Bacterial or fungal overgrowth cause inflammation and clog your plumbing, making it difficult to absorb nutrients.

- Supplement your diet daily with a probiotic containing 3 to 20 billion viable cells of *Lactobacillus* and *Bifidobacterium* species.

Assess Your Level of Inflammation

If your signs and symptoms indicate inflammation, you should try to obtain laboratory testing to assess your level of oxidative stress and systemic inflammation (see chapter 4). The more objective information you have as therapeutic targets, the better your treatment management will be. Don't just guess when determining your treatment regime. Be as scientific about your therapy as possible. My favorite supplements for reducing oxidative stress and inflammation are alpha-lipoic acid, curcumin, fish oil, N-acetyl cysteine, taurine, and milk thistle.

Check for Good Hormonal Regulation

Sometimes, no matter how sound your nutritional program is, achieving good skeletal health may require hormone replacement therapy. Ask your doctor if hormonal therapy, preferably in the form of bioidentical hormones, would be useful to reduce your fracture risk.

Rule Out Toxins

If you have any concerns about heavy metal toxicity, check with your doctor about getting some laboratory testing.

Supplement with Body- and Bone-Building Nutrients

Whey protein (20 grams/day) will help you increase your IGF-1 level and build both muscle and bone mass. (If your stomach doesn't like all that protein at once, you can split up 20 grams into two shakes with 10 grams of whey protein in each shake.) Not only will this help to raise your body's antioxidant levels of glutathione, the lactoferrin and lactoferricin in whey also will help to limit the growth of bad bacteria, such as *H. pylori*, in your GI tract.

In animal and cell culture studies, whey and its milk basic protein component have been shown to stimulate osteoblasts (Takada, Aoe, and Kumegawa 1996), suppress osteoclast-mediated bone resorption, and enhance bone strength (Takada et al. 1997). Moreover, a study of healthy adult women showed that supplementing with whey's basic protein fraction significantly increased their BMD (Yamamura et al 2002). A shake made with whey, fruit, and your choice of other supplements is a refreshing, nutritious midafternoon snack. Also, nutrition companies are selling high-quality powdered supplement mixes and meal replacement mixes that can make your life easier and your afternoon snacking healthier.

If you are low on energy, acetyl-L-carnitine (2g/day), biotin, alpha-lipoic acid, and coenzyme Q10 will help to supply your cells with energy. These supplements will reduce fatigue and help you build muscle.

If you have osteoporosis but your bone resorption marker (NTX, CTX, or DPD) is normal, make sure your doctor orders a test for the bone formation marker osteocalcin. This will indicate if you need to work hard on stimulating your osteoblasts to form new bone. Nutrients such as vitamin K, milk basic protein, and whey protein, in addition to ensuring that your body is not acidic (check your urine pH), are most important for bone formation. When you succeed in stimulating osteoblastic activity, it will be reflected by the normalization of your blood osteocalcin levels. You might also want to try using the selective kinase response modulators (SKRMs), berberine and/or rho-iso-alpha acids (RIAA), the latter from hops (see chapter 4).

Exercise!

Exercise regularly to your own capacity, and it will help you maintain a healthy body and strong bones. For safety, check with your doctor and make sure he or she clears you for starting an exercise program. If you are having musculoskeletal pain or have physical restrictions, a physical therapist can help you get started. Once you're capable, a certified personal trainer can help you achieve the next level of fitness.

Once you feel comfortable on your own, exercise at least three to four times a week either at a gym or at home. If you get bored with your program, get excited about some new exercises. This is the fun part. Enjoy it. Meet some new people. Experience how good it feels to take in deep breaths and move your body.

Consider Medications Carefully

If your BMD is below -2.5, and especially if you have fractured, you should talk with your doctor about using a medication. Weigh all considerations; your decision should be made strictly from the information that pertains to you, and not from the dogma of any one therapeutic specialty. New drugs are constantly being designed, so if your doctor is considering an osteoporosis medication for you, make sure to ask about any new ones that may be available. For example, the drug odanacatib is currently in clinical trials. Odanacatib differs from bisphosphonates in that it can increase BMD not by killing the osteoclasts, but by inhibiting their release of a bone-degrading enzyme.

If you're a small-boned individual and your BMD is low, your T-score may just be normal for you. Check out some biomarkers first before consenting too quickly to a prescription. If your bone resorption marker is normal, your vitamin D is normal, you don't have gastrointestinal problems or gluten sensitivity, and you're not on any bone-draining medications and don't have any other risk factors, then your low BMD may just be normal for you.

Monitor and Constantly Tweak

That is all there is to it. You're on your own (with the help of your doctor, of course). For the first year or two, you and your doctor will need to use regular laboratory testing to monitor your progress. During this time you'll be using various test results to tweak your nutritional supplementation program or, possibly, begin or alter your use of a medication. Eventually, however, you'll settle into a program that suits your needs. You have the tools you need. Go for it!

CHAPTER TEN

Bone Pearls

Once in a while, when I go tracking in the forest, I come across a scattering of bones, the decaying last remnants of a creature's existence here on earth. It's not death that I see in these bones but a silent record of the animal's life and proof of its untold transformations. If you study these final bastions of life closely enough, you'll notice subtle signs within their cortex, trabeculae, marrow, and overall structure—signs that tell of past feast or famine, growth or decline, health or disease. Like ancient talismans etched with cryptic writings, they tell stories if you know how to read them. Even in death, bones continue to resonate with all the essence that once surrounded them. I consider them stunning, sacred, white pearls of encapsulated history.

Our wilderness trek is about to end, but your journey for skeletal health is just beginning. You've experienced the dangers of the forest, fraught with inflammatory fires, dysbiotic quagmires, microbial goblins, and toxic waterways. Now that you're aware of the dangers of the forest and how to circumvent them, you can find your way. You have the information to forge ahead and improve your skeletal health. There may be setbacks; there certainly will be improvements. Take one step at a time and keep going. You are writing your own story, your own script—only now it is one of renewal.

CLINICAL BONE PEARLS

Clinical pearls are practical tips used by doctors to help solve problems or improve therapeutic outcomes. You've learned a lot of facts about the inner workings of your skeleton. Now here are some final pearls for the rest of your odyssey. Think of them as gifts from all the beings that lived in and walked through the forest before you.

Start Your Day "Green"

Along with a wholesome breakfast, start your day with a green drink. Many nutrition companies offer powdered blends of dried fruits, vegetables, and grasses that are reconstituted with water or juice to make a powerfully healing drink packed with vitamins, minerals, and enzymes. A tablespoon of concentrated greens each morning will help cleanse, alkalinize, and rejuvenate your body—a great way to start your day.

Drink a Recovery Shake Immediately After You Exercise

Get the most out of your whey protein shakes by drinking one within fifteen to twenty minutes after you exercise. That's when your muscles are starving for nutrition (carbohydrates and protein). I recommend that your postworkout recovery drink have a ratio of carbohydrate to protein between 2:1 and 4:1, depending on the workout. Consuming from 0.4 g/kg to 0.8 g/kg of carbohydrates and 0.2 g/kg to 0.4 g/kg of protein within half an hour after exercising will optimize your routine's anabolic benefit.

A workout like weight lifting, which is geared toward building muscle strength, requires more protein to repair and build muscles and less carbohydrate. Thus, a carbohydrate to protein ratio of 1:2 would be the most beneficial. Conversely, a workout focused on endurance, such as walking or running, calls for more carbohydrate; thus a 4:1 ratio to recharge muscles with energy is the best. It's important to recharge your muscles as soon as possible after a workout. This is a great way to battle the sarcopenia so commonly associated with osteoporosis, and it gives you the energy you need to stick with your regular exercise routine.

There are many whey-based, powdered supplement mixes or meal-replacement mixes that can make your life a bit easier. Find one with a carbohydrate to protein ratio that fits your needs and has a taste you like, measure out what you want into a large-mouthed container, and take it to the gym with you. After your workout, add water to the container, shake it, and drink it down.

Core-Strengthening Exercises Help Reduce Fractures

Strengthening your core, or trunk, muscles helps reduce fracture risk by improving balance and preventing falls. Core exercises (on the floor or with physio balls) also stabilize the spine and specifically help to reduce spinal compression fractures. Because the spinal vertebrae are the bones most vulnerable to fracture in osteoporosis, it certainly makes sense to include core strengthening in your regular exercise routine.

Seek Chiropractic Treatment for Pain from Compression Fractures

Spinal compression fractures can be very painful, and a chiropractor can help. If you have sustained a compression fracture and are experiencing residual pain, muscle spasms, or restricted motion long after the fracture has healed, gentle chiropractic spinal manipulation and soft-tissue rehabilitation techniques can provide relief.

Supplement with Amino Acids to Aid Hormone Production

A catabolic osteoporotic physiology is intensely stressed and requires a constant source of amino acids for tissue repair and the balanced production of hormones. In this stressful situation, it is the production of hormones that suffers most. Daily supplementation with 5 grams of an amino acid blend for six months to a year (or longer if necessary) will help your body to cope with this need.

Make Krill Oil Your Friend

Antarctic krill (shrimplike crustaceans) are loaded with omega-3-rich oils (DHA and EPA) and a very powerful antioxidant called astaxanthin. Krill oil will not only help to reduce cholesterol and triglycerides and increase HDLs, it will also reduce hs-CRP, which is important for decreasing fracture risk. Krill oil is also capable of reducing reactive oxygen species (ROS), also known as free radicals, better than most other antioxidants available.

If You Can Do Only a Few Things to Improve Your Bone Health, Do These...

Make reducing excessive osteoclastic activity your primary goal for beating osteoporosis, especially if your bone resorption marker is elevated. As you are now aware, this process can be complex and it often involves multiple therapeutic approaches to reduce inflammation and oxidative stress, improve gut health, eliminate toxins, and so forth. But if I had to emphasize just a few vital steps for reducing bone resorption and improving skeletal health, they would be the following:

- Promote neutral body pH by eating lots of fruits and vegetables, and if necessary, supplement with potassium to maintain urine pH above 6.6.

- Normalize gut function with the following

  - Fiber such as arabinogalactan (which is also a food for good bacteria)

  - Probiotics

  - Digestive enzymes if needed

- Go gluten free if your antibody biomarkers are elevated

- Supplement daily with a multivitamin-mineral, and make sure you're getting 1,200 mg/day calcium, 600 mg/day magnesium, 2,000 IU/day of vitamin D, 1 mg/day vitamin K, alpha-lipoic acid, N-acetyl cysteine, milk thistle, possibly berberine, and fish oil or flaxseed.

- Make a shake using whey protein (20 g/day) for your afternoon snack.

- Exercise (three to four days a week).

Milk Basic Protein Increases Osteocalcin

Supplementing with milk basic protein was shown to prevent bone loss in women aged sixty-five to eighty-six in the Nakanojo Study (Park et al. 2007). If you are osteoporotic and have sarcopenia, and especially if your osteocalcin (bone formation biomarker) is low, consider supplementing with milk basic protein.

Treat Yourself to Some Bone-Building Muffins

Jeannette Bessinger, a nutrition educator and coauthor of *Simple Food for Busy Families* (Bessinger and Yablon-Brenner 2009), has at my request whipped up a batch of good-tasting and good-for-you muffins. With everything in them to make your skeleton healthy, these muffins are a convenient way to maintain good nutrition for your bones throughout the day.

Jeannette ingeniously came up with this recipe, which is loaded with calcium and magnesium, and many other bone-enriching ingredients. These include xylitol (the bone-building sweetener with a low glycemic index), blackstrap molasses (high in vitamin K, calcium, and potassium), coconut oil (high in medium-chain triglycerides, easy to digest, packed with energy, and very healthy for your gut), tasty alkaline vegetables (high in fiber), and flaxseed (for its phytoestrogens and to reduce inflammation). Adding figs or prunes boosts levels of calcium, magnesium, potassium, antioxidants, and vitamin K, and the walnuts provide a special osteoblast-stimulating bioflavonoid called myricetin. You just can't find any tastier bone-healthy muffins than these. They can be frozen, so you can always have them on hand for a snack or to take to work. Make a batch and enjoy!

Bone-Healthy Muffin Recipe

Ingredients

2½ cups whole-wheat pastry flour or gluten-free baking flour from garbanzo beans

½ cup wheat bran

½ cup whey protein powder

¼ cup ground flaxseeds

1 teaspoon baking soda

¼ teaspoon baking powder

2 teaspoons cinnamon

½ teaspoon nutmeg

3 eggs

1 cup xylitol

¾ cup virgin coconut oil

¼ cup blackstrap molasses

¼ cup orange or apple juice concentrate

2 cups pureed zucchini (unpeeled)

1 cup grated sweet potato (peeled)

1 cup dark chocolate chips (grain-sweetened is fine unless you have celiac disease)

1 cup chopped walnuts (optional)

Directions

Preheat the oven to 325º F and line 24 muffin cups with paper liners.

In a large bowl, combine the flour, bran, whey powder, flaxseeds, baking soda, baking powder, cinnamon, and nutmeg and stir until well mixed.

Beat the eggs in a mixer for about 2 minutes, until light and foamy. Add the xylitol, coconut oil, molasses, and juice concentrate and mix on low speed just until combined. Stir in the zucchini and sweet potato.

Gently fold the egg mixture into the dry ingredients until thoroughly blended, then add the chocolate chips and walnuts and stir once or twice.

Scoop the dough into the prepared muffin tin, filling each cup about three-quarters full. Bake for about 20 minutes, until a toothpick inserted in the center of a muffin comes out clean, then cool on a wire rack.

For moister muffins, use 1½ cups zucchini pureed to applesauce consistency in a food processor (about 2 small zucchinis). Instead of chocolate chips, you can use 1 cup of dried figs or prunes. Dice them or chop them in a food processor until you have small, raisin-size chunks. (I prefer the muffins with figs.)

Yield: 2 dozen muffins

Supplement with Creatine and D-Ribose for Muscle Mass and Energy

Creatine, an amino acid complex, and *D-ribose*, a natural sugar, are produced in your body and are essential for the production of *adenosine triphosphate* (ATP; cell energy). As we age, the levels of creatine and D-ribose within our bodies fall and our energy suffers. If you're having difficulty putting on muscle even with a good resistance-training program, try supplementing with creatine and D-ribose. They will help to increase your muscle mass, strength, and power. Where there's muscle mass, bone mass will follow. Where there's strength, there are fewer falls. And where there's power, there is a fuller experience of life.

Stay Positive

There is a lot to be said for the mind-body connection. Stay positive, throw any negative thoughts you may have to the wind, put your heart and soul into this journey, and never give up. With this attitude, your health and the world as a whole will benefit.

SEEING HEALTH DIFFERENTLY

I hope your eyes are now opened to a unique and valuable way of looking at skeletal health. Your vision has certainly been sharpened, and you've been made more keenly aware of the subtleties of physiology that unfold as either health or disease. You now know that your skeleton is full of individual players, and to keep or make you healthy, they must all coalesce as a whole. As biological entities, each player relies on the whole body for physiological teamwork, intimate partnerships, and complex backup mechanisms, and each often multitasks between the immune and skeletal systems.

In truth, no single skeletal element functions independently or has just one job—just as no single member of a forest community lives in isolation separated from the rest of the forest's inhabitants. Each of our skeletal elements intricately and economically holds us together in multiple ways. But just as their fine-tuning provides us with functional balance, so too can their disruption lead to crumbling. Any element's failure—no matter how distant from the skeleton—can be a source of structural failure. And so too can any element's realignment and restoration be a source of structural healing.

The approach this book offers has the ability to take you to a level of well-being far beyond what would be possible through the use of medication alone. When treating your osteoporosis, you no longer have to simply settle for harder bones. By putting effort into regaining your health, the whole quality of your life will prosper, and your efforts will be repaid in comfort, capability, longevity, and happiness many times over. Your eyes will never look at a forest—any forest—the same way, ever again.

Appendix

Key Nutrients for Bone Health

Calcium. This mineral is vital for skeletal mineralization, blood clotting, conduction of nerve impulses, buffering of acidic blood, enzyme activity, and muscle contractions.

- **Deficiency signs and symptoms:** Bone loss, periodontal disease, tooth decay, and muscle spasms.

- **Biomarkers**
  Comprehensive metabolic panel (CMP): The level of calcium in your blood can be obtained through a CMP. If elevated, it may indicate an overactive parathyroid gland or a malignancy. If low, it may indicate that you are not getting enough calcium or that you have a malabsorption problem, a magnesium deficiency, or an insufficient secretion of the parathyroid hormone (PTH) from your parathyroid glands.
  Hair: Interpretation of calcium status is difficult with hair analysis, but early detection of low bone density caused by endocrine disease (hyperparathyroidism or hyperthyroidism) can be seen when there is a significant increase in the calcium level of hair (Miekeley et al. 2001).

- **Laboratory correlates**
  Vitamin D [25(OH)D]: If your calcium is low, it may mean insufficient vitamin D.
  Magnesium: Low blood calcium can be due to a deficiency of magnesium.
  Albumin: Low albumin levels may be due to low blood calcium

levels or to overall poor nutrition.

Celiac profile: Low calcium can indicate the malabsorption of celiac disease.

Anemia: If low calcium and anemia are found, it is important to test for celiac disease.

- **Dietary sources:** Dairy products, figs, vegetables (especially kale, broccoli, bok choy, collards, mustard greens, and turnip greens), sea vegetables, bean sprouts, spinach, teff (a nongluten grain), nuts, seeds, beans, and tofu.

- **Supplementation:** Microcrystalline hydroxyapatite complex, calcium citrate, or calcium citrate/malate are the best sources for supplemental calcium. Adult daily intake should be 1,200 to 1,500 mg/day. Your calcium to phosphorus dietary ratio should be 1:1 and not exceed 2:1.

Phosphorus. This mineral is important for energy, enzyme activity, muscle contraction, and nerve contractions.

- **Deficiency signs and symptoms:** Malnutrition.

- **Biomarkers:** *CMP.* If elevated, it may indicate kidney disease or genetic disorders. Elevated phosphorus may also be seen with bisphosphonate use. If low, it may indicate malabsorption, hyperparathyroid, or genetic disorders.

- **Laboratory correlates**
Vitamin D: Low phosphorus may indicate vitamin D insufficiency.
Calcium: Blood calcium levels will be affected by fluctuations in blood phosphorus.
PTH: Abnormal phosphorus levels can mean a parathyroid gland disorder.

- **Dietary sources:** Most foods, especially dairy, cereals, eggs, and meat.

- **Supplementation:** Phosphorus is abundant in most foods and usually unnecessary to supplement. In fact, the Western diet is often too high in acid-producing phosphorus. Keep your dietary ratio of phosphorus to calcium at 1:1. High-phosphorus diets lead to metabolic acidosis and calcium loss.

Magnesium. This is one of the most important nutrients in your body. It is vital for cell energy metabolism, nerve conduction, cell membrane integrity, electrolyte balance, and the proper functioning of over three hundred enzymes. Deficiency reduces osteoblast bone formation and increases osteoclast bone resorption. Magnesium is necessary for release of the hormone calcitonin from the thyroid gland, and for the production of parathyroid hormone. Both hormones are necessary for bone health.

- **Deficiency signs and symptoms:** Muscle spasms, skin twitching below the eye, constipation, hypertension, rapid heart rate, arrhythmias, depression, fatigue, asthma, muscle weakness, irritability, and hypersensitive skin.

- **Biomarkers:** *Red blood cell (RBC) magnesium.* Only whole-blood magnesium levels accurately reflect total body levels. Serum magnesium is not a good indicator of total body level.

- **Laboratory correlates**
  Calcium (blood): Inadequate magnesium may cause low serum calcium.
  Potassium: Low serum potassium can correlate to low magnesium levels.
  Vitamin D (active vitamin D [$1,25(OH)_2D$]: This form of vitamin D may be low when total magnesium levels are inadequate.
  Anemia: Low magnesium can lead to anemia (seen on CBC).
  PTH: Low magnesium levels can elevate parathyroid hormone levels.
  Osteocalcin (bone formation marker): Inadequate bone formation, as reflected by low osteocalcin, may be a consequence of inadequate magnesium.
  Hs-CRP (C-reactive protein): Low magnesium can increases the pro-inflammatory cytokines (IL-6 and TNF) and would be reflected as elevated levels of hs-CRP.

- **Dietary sources:** Legumes, whole grains, broccoli, green leafy vegetables, animal protein, seeds (especially pumpkin), nuts, and, yes, chocolate.

- **Supplementation:** 600 to 750 mg/day may be optimal for osteoporosis. Keep your calcium to magnesium intake ratio balanced at approximately 2:1. Use magnesium ascorbate, aspartate, gluconate, or malate. Avoid magnesium oxide and carbonate. Note that excess magnesium can give you loose stools.

Zinc. Zinc deficiency is common. It is often seen in malabsorption syndromes, alcoholism, and with long-term intense exercise. Zinc deficiency contributes to bone loss and is linked to low BMD and reduced IGF-1. The enzyme that converts the thyroid hormone T4 to the active form, T3, is zinc dependent, and therefore zinc deficiency may lead to low thyroid function.

- **Deficiency signs and symptoms:** White spots on fingernails or chronic finger infections along the nail bed, in addition to a decreased sense of taste or smell. Frequent colds, poor wound healing, infections, chronic sickness, impotence, and altered vision can all be signs or symptoms of zinc deficiency.

- **Biomarkers:** *RBC zinc test, zinc taste test.* Note that the zinc taste test's validity has not been thoroughly researched.

- **Laboratory correlates**
  Thyroid profile: Low thyroid function may be seen with low levels of zinc.
  IGF-1: Low IGF-1 may be due to low zinc levels.
  Alkaline phosphatase: Low alkaline phosphatase can mean low levels of zinc.
  Testosterone: Low testosterone has been associated with low levels of zinc.

- **Dietary sources:** Seafood (especially oysters), beef, chicken, liver, spinach, nuts, and seeds.

- **Supplementation:** If deficient, 15 to 25 mg/day of zinc and no more than 40 mg/day. Copper, at 2.5 mg/day, should accompany zinc supplementation (the ideal zinc to copper ratio is 7.5:1). Use zinc picolinate, zinc glycinate, or zinc citrate. Avoid zinc oxide.

Potassium. High dietary intake and supplementation with potassium will rectify chronic low-level metabolic acidosis and concomitant urine calcium losses. Adequate potassium is important for overall acid-base balance.

- **Deficiency signs and symptoms:** None specific, but high sodium (salt) intake increases potassium excretion and may increase your blood pressure.

- **Biomarkers:** *Comprehensive metabolic panel.*

- **Laboratory correlates**

  Urine pH: If your morning urine pH level is consistently below 6.0, it may indicate that you are low in potassium.

  Magnesium: Low magnesium and low potassium often correlate.

- **Dietary sources:** Fruits, vegetables, and beans.

- **Supplementation:** Potassium bicarbonate or citrate, 500 to 2,000 mg/day to reduce the acidity of your body (as seen in persistently low urine pH). Note: It is preferable to obtain potassium through dietary sources, but if body acidity remains low, supplementation may be necessary. Total daily intake of potassium should be approximately 4,000 to 5,000 mg. Caution: Supplementation of potassium when taking ACE inhibitors, angiotension receptor blockers, or potassium-sparing diuretics, can result in hyperkalemia (high blood potassium levels) and heart arrhythmias. You don't want to do that. Check this with your doctor.

Boron. Supplemental boron may help to increase BMD by increasing estrogen levels in postmenopausal women. Note: If you have a cancer that is estrogen sensitive, such as breast, uterine, or ovarian cancer, boron supplementation should be avoided.

- **Deficiency signs and symptoms:** None specific.

- **Biomarkers:** *Serum* (blood) or *urine analysis.*

- **Laboratory correlates:** *Estrogen:* Low estradiol may indicate low boron.

- **Dietary sources:** Prunes, grapes, peanuts, pecans, apples, beans, and vegetables.

- **Supplementation:** Boron citrate 3 to 20 mg/day.

Manganese. Deficiency of this trace mineral is linked to osteoporosis.

- **Deficiency signs and symptoms:** None specific.

- **Biomarkers:** *Red blood cell analysis.*

- **Laboratory correlates:** *Superoxide dismutase:* Low.

- **Dietary sources:** Nuts, seeds, legumes, green vegetables, whole grains, and tea.

- **Supplementation:** 5 mg/day.

Copper. This mineral is important for enzyme activity and acts as a catalytic agent during biochemical processes involved in the formation of bone. Deficiency is rare.

- **Deficiency signs and symptoms:** Anemia, elevated cholesterol.

- **Biomarkers:** *Serum ceruloplasmin, white blood cells* (WBCs) in CBC (low WBCs may indicate a need for copper), *red blood cell analysis.*

- **Laboratory correlates**
  Superoxide dismutase: Low.
  Bone resorption biomarkers: In osteoporotic individuals, low levels may be due to copper deficiency (Kawada et al. 2006).

- **Dietary sources:** Organ meats, seafood, eggs, nuts, seeds, wheat bran, grains, and cocoa.

- **Supplementation:** 2.5 to 5 mg/day.

Silica. This trace mineral is important for the development of strong collagen fibers. When silica is deficient, bone collagen structural cross-links develop poorly and lead to reduced bone strength.

- **Deficiency signs and symptoms:** None specific.

- **Biomarkers:** None.

- **Laboratory correlates:** None.

- **Dietary sources:** Outer layer of grains (bran), skin (rind) and fiber from fruits and vegetables, unfiltered drinking water, and horsetail grass tea.

- **Supplementation:** 25 to 40 mg/day.

Vitamin A. This is necessary for bone health, but excess vitamin A (retinol) intake correlates to low BMD.

- **Deficiency signs and symptoms:** Bumpy skin on back of arms; dry, flaky skin.

- **Biomarkers:** *Plasma retinol, plasma carotene.*

- **Laboratory correlates:** None.

- **Dietary sources:** Retinol from meat. Beta-carotene from orange and yellow fruits and vegetables and dark green leafy vegetables.

- **Supplementation:** Excess vitamin A (retinol) can suppress osteoblastic activity, increase osteoclastic bone resorption, and interfere with vitamin D metabolism. One study (Feskanich et al. 2002) linked vitamin A intake to increased fracture risk, although a more recent study (Barker et al. 2005) found no such association. Just to be on the safe side, I recommend not exceeding 8,000 IU/day of supplemental vitamin A. And if your diet includes dairy products and plenty of fruits and vegetables, supplementing may not be necessary at all.

Vitamin B Complex. Vitamins B_2, B_6, B_{12}, and folic acid are all important for reducing homocysteine if it is elevated. Reducing elevated homocysteine with the supplementation of these vitamins will help reduce fracture risk.

Vitamin B_2 (Riboflavin): This vitamin is important for tissue respiration and enzyme activity.

- **Deficiency signs and symptoms:** Celiac disease, cracks at the edges of the mouth, glossitis (inflammation or infection of the tongue).

- **Biomarkers:** Not commonly assayed.

- **Laboratory correlates:** *Homocysteine:* Elevated.

- **Dietary sources:** Milk, meat, eggs, nuts, and green vegetables.

- **Supplementation:** Take 25 mg/day to reduce homocysteine.

Vitamin B_6 (Pyridoxine). Vitamin B_6 is necessary to produce hydrochloric acid for good digestion and calcium absorption. It's also important for vitamin K to work well.

- **Deficiency signs and symptoms:** Premenstrual symptoms, carpal tunnel syndrome, cheilosis (cracks in the corners of the mouth).

- **Biomarkers:** *Serum pyridoxine* (not commonly assayed).

- **Laboratory correlates:** *Homocysteine.* Elevated.

- **Dietary sources:** Meat, eggs, nuts, and grains.

- **Supplementation:** Take 50 to 250 mg/day to reduce homocysteine.

Vitamin B$_{12}$ (Cyanocobalamin). Vitamin B$_{12}$ is important for nerve sheath health and red blood cell production. Vitamin B$_{12}$ deficiency is common when stomach acidity is low, and with the use of proton pump inhibitors (PPIs).

- **Deficiency signs and symptoms:** Depression, numbness and tingling, ataxia (poor muscular coordination), poor memory, hearing loss, weakness, glossitis (tongue inflammation), a burning sensation in the mouth.

- **Biomarkers**
  Serum cobalamin (B$_{12}$): This is the most common marker used by physicians to detect frank deficiency, but it is not sensitive for assessing inadequate B$_{12}$ levels.
  Serum methylmalonic acid.
  Urine organic acid methylmalonate.

- **Laboratory correlates:** *Homocysteine.* Elevated.

- **Dietary sources:** Formed by microorganisms in the gut; also meat, fish, and liver.

- **Supplementation:** Take 1,000 mcg/day to reduce homocysteine.

Folate. This is important for normal red blood cell development.

- **Deficiency signs and symptoms:** Gingivitis, cheilosis, glossitis.

- **Biomarkers**
  Red blood cell folacin (folic acid).
  CBC: Mean corpuscular volume (MCV) may be increased.

- **Laboratory correlates:** *Homocysteine.* Elevated.

- **Dietary sources:** Green leafy vegetables.

- **Supplementation:** Take 400 mcg/day to reduce homocysteine.

Vitamin C. This important antioxidant maintains structural integrity of collagen fibers, boosts energy metabolism, and enhances immune function.

- **Deficiency signs and symptoms:** Fatigue, bleeding and swollen gums, loose teeth, bluish gums, small hemorrhages around the base of hair shafts.

- **Biomarkers:** None reliable.

- **Laboratory correlates**
  Hs-CRP: Elevated hs-CRP can be reduced with increased vitamin C.
  Lipid peroxides: Elevated lipid peroxides can be reduced with vitamin C.

- **Dietary sources:** Fruits and vegetables, especially citrus fruits.

- **Supplementation:** 1,000 to 2,000 mg/day.

Vitamin D. This vitamin comes in two forms: vitamin D_3 and vitamin D_2. It ensures adequate blood calcium levels by increasing calcium absorption from the gut. If calcium intake is insufficient and blood calcium levels drop, PTH from the parathyroid gland is released, and more vitamin D (if in adequate supply) is activated. This activated vitamin D stimulates osteoblasts to release RANKL, a chemical messenger that activates osteoclastic bone resorption in order to access calcium stores. Production of PTH depends on adequate magnesium. When supplementing with vitamin D, always include adequate calcium and magnesium. Optimal vitamin D levels improve absorption of calcium, improve strength, and reduce fracture risk. In addition, this vitamin helps to decrease the risk of cancer, diabetes, and heart disease.

- **Deficiency signs and symptoms:** Osteoporosis, bone pain, sternum and shin bones sore to the touch, muscle weakness, psoriatic (pitted) nails.

- **Biomarkers**
  Vitamin D (inactive form, 25-hydroxyvitamin D [25(OH)D]): This is the most important form to assess. If you have osteoporosis and your vitamin D is low (below 35 ng/ml), your levels should be measured twice a year until adequate levels are reached.
  Vitamin D (active form, 1,25-dihydroxyvitamin D [1,25(OH)$_2$D]).

- **Laboratory correlates:** *PTH* (parathyroid hormone). If your vitamin D level is found to be low, your PTH should be slightly elevated. If your PTH is low or even normal, it may be an indication of magnesium deficiency. This condition is referred to as functional hypoparathyroidism because magnesium is required for the production of PTH.

- **Dietary sources:** Sunlight (ultraviolet B radiation) exposure (5 to 10 minutes/day 2 to 3 times/week), cod liver oil, oily fish, fortified milk, and fortified orange juice.

- **Supplementation:** 2,000 IU/day or more may be necessary to maintain sufficient levels. Note: when taking high doses of vitamin D, it is important to complement its action with supplemental vitamin K unless you are currently taking a blood-thinning medication.

Vitamin K. This is crucial for blood coagulation and bone formation. Deficiency is associated with low BMD and increased fracture risk. Vitamins K and D work in concert. Vitamin D increases calcium absorption from the gut, and vitamin K prevents calcium loss in the urine. In bone, vitamin D stimulates osteoblasts to produce the protein osteocalcin, which is so important for mineralization, and vitamin K activates the osteocalcin. Inadequate vitamin K contributes to soft tissue calcification.

- **Deficiency signs and symptoms:** Bruising, small areas of bleeding under the skin, incidental vessel calcifications noted on X-rays of the chest or spine.

- **Biomarkers**
  Prothrombin time (PT): This is the most commonly used test to assess for vitamin K deficiency, but it is not a sensitive marker.
  Serum phylloquinone: This test is also of limited clinical use as it reflects only recent dietary intake of vitamin K.
  PIVKA-II (protein induced by vitamin K absence): This is a more sensitive marker than PT.
  Undercarboxylated osteocalcin: The best test—a functional marker for vitamin K.

- **Laboratory correlates**
  Calcification of vessels (noted incidentally on X-ray): Although this is not a true laboratory correlate, it can be a useful sign of the need for vitamin K.

Calcium (urine): High calcium loss in the urine can be reduced with vitamin K.

- **Dietary sources:** K$_1$ (phylloquinone) is found in dark green vegetables, such as asparagus, kale, broccoli, spinach, and seaweed. The other major form, K$_2$ (menaquinone), is made by bacteria and is found in meat, liver, and milk.

- **Supplementation:** Daily reference intake (DRI) is 1.5 µg per kilogram of body weight per day, but it is thought that at least 200 to 500 µg/day may be necessary for optimal osteocalcin activity (Vermeer 2004). For osteoporosis, 1 mg/day is recommended for general support, but very high doses (45 mg/day) of K$_2$ have been used to treat osteoporosis in Japan (Shiraki et al. 2000). The MK-7 form of K$_2$ appears to be the superior supplemental form. Warning: If taking an anticoagulant such as coumadin (Warfarin) or acenocoumarol (Sinthrome), it has been advised not to exceed 100 µg/day of vitamin K.

Essential Fatty Acids (EFAs). The EFAs, alpha-linolenic acid (omega-3) and linoleic acid (omega-6), are long-chain polyunsaturated fatty acids that must be obtained through your diet or by supplementation. They are important for healthy cell membranes and have a primary role in your immune system's regulation of inflammation. The conversion of linolenic acid to EPA and DHA (other forms of omega-3, which are also important for disease prevention), and linoleic acid to other important fatty acids, is through the enzyme delta-6-desaturase. The function of this enzyme is adversely affected by low levels of zinc, vitamin B$_6$, and magnesium. Omega-3 deficiency is common and is linked to heart disease, cancer, insulin resistance, depression, accelerated aging, diabetes, Alzheimer's, and other diseases.

- **Deficiency signs and symptoms:** Thin, lifeless, low-luster hair; bumpy skin on back of arms; seborrhea at the folds at the edge of the nose; fatigue; dry mucous membranes; eczema; joint pain; poor memory or concentration; and depression.

- **Biomarkers:** *Essential fatty acid profiles.* Available through specialty labs.

- **Laboratory correlates**
  Triglycerides and LDL cholesterol: When these are increased, it may indicate a need for EFAs.

HDL cholesterol: Low HDL indicates a need for EFAs.

Calcium (urine): High loss of calcium in urine can indicate a need for EFAs.

Hs-CRP: When hs-CRP is elevated, EFA supplementation is indicated.

- **Dietary sources:** Fish (cold-water fish, such as sardines, mackerel, salmon, bluefish, and herring); krill, canola, and hemp oil; walnuts; and seeds, such as chia, pumpkin, flax, and sunflower.

- **Supplementation:** 1,000 to 2,000 mg/day. Use a balance of fish or krill oil for omega-3 fats, and borage, evening primrose, or black currant seed oil for omega-6 fats. Hemp oil and flaxseed have a good ratio of omega-3 to omega-6 fats.

Amino Acids. These are the building blocks of protein. They are vital to your bone health and overall health. They are important for the growth and repair of all tissues, including bone collagen. Amino acids also provide the foundation for all hormones, messenger cytokines, and enzymes involved in each step of the bone remodeling process. People with osteoporosis are commonly deficient in amino acids, especially when there is malabsorption or poor digestion. The amino acid lysine, found in meat, dairy, and eggs, is particularly important for bone health. If you have osteoporosis, and especially if you are a vegetarian, make sure you supplement your diet with 500 mg/day of lysine.

- **Deficiency signs and symptoms:** Weight loss, depression, fatigue, and low hormone levels.

- **Biomarkers:** *Plasma and urine amino acid profiles.* Available from specialty labs.

- **Laboratory correlates:** *Albumin.* Low.

- **Dietary sources:** Dairy (especially whey protein), eggs, meat, soy, and legumes.

- **Supplementation:** Whey protein or an amino acid blend.

Note: Much of the information in this section was obtained from Werbach and Moss 1999; Pizzorno and Murray 2000; Jellin et al. 2006; and Lord and Bralley 2008.

Resources

COMPANIES WITH QUALITY NUTRITIONAL PRODUCTS

Note: This list is not all-inclusive. It is meant to be used only as a starting point.

AOR (Advanced Orthomolecular Research)
800-387-0177
www.aor.ca

Biogenesis Nutraceuticals
866-272-0500
www.bio-genesis.com

Biotics Research
800-231-5777
www.bioticsresearch.com

Crayhon Research
777-823-5333
www.crayhonresearch.com

Designs for Health
800-367-4325
www.designsforhealth.com

Doctor Greens
603-447-9282
www.doctorgreens.com

Innate Response Formulas
800-634-6342
www.innateresponse.com

Metagenics
800-692-9400
www.metagenics.com

NBI (Nutritional Biochemistry, Inc.)
800-624-1416
www.nbihealth.com

Nordic Naturals
800-662-2544
www.nordicnaturals.com

Perque
800-525-7372
www.perque.com

Pharmax
800-538-8274
www.pharmaxllc.com

PhytoPharmica
800-376-7789
www.phytopharmica.com

ProThera
888-488-2488
www.protherainc.com

Pure Encapsulations
800-753-2277
www.purecaps.com

Standard Process
800-848-5061
www.standardprocess.com

Theramedix
866-998-4372
www.theramedix.net

Thorne Research
208-263-1337
www.thorne.com

Vital Nutrients
888-328-9922
www.vitalnutrients.net

Xymogen
877-377-9320
www.xymogen.com

SPECIALTY LABORATORIES

Note: This list in not all-inclusive. It is meant to be used only as a starting point.

Doctor's Data
800-323-2784
www.doctor'sdata.com

Diagnos-Techs
800-878-3787
www.diagnostechs.com

Genova Diagnostics
800-522-4762
www.genovadiagnostics.com

Great Plains Laboratory
800-288-0383
www.greatplainslaboratory.com

Meridian Valley Laboratory
425-271-8689
www.meridianvalleylab.com

Metametrix Clinical Laboratory
800-221-4640
www.metametrix.com

SpectraCell Laboratories
800-227-5227
www.spectracell.com

US BioTek Laboratories
206-365-1256
www.usbiotek.com

References

Alexandersen, P., A. Toussaint, C. Christiansen, J. P. Devogelaer, C. Roux, J. Fechtenbaum, et al. 2001. Ipriflavone in the treatment of postmeno-pausal osteoporosis: A randomized controlled trial. *Journal of the American Medical Association* 285(11):1482-1488.

Anderson, G. L., M. Limacher, R. A. Assaf, T. Bassford, S. A. Beresford, H. Black, et al. 2004. Effects of conjugated equine estrogen in postmenopausal women with hysterectomy: The Women's Health Initiative randomized controlled trial. *Journal of the American Medical Association* 291(14):1701-1712.

Arrieta, M. C., L. Bistritz, and J. B. Meddings. 2006. Alterations in intestinal permeability. *Gut* 55(10):1512-1520.

Bagger, Y. Z., H. B. Rasmussen, P. Alexandersen, T. Werge, C. Christiansen, L. B. Tankó, et al. 2007. Links between cardiovascular disease and osteo-porosis in postmenopausal women: Serum lipids or atherosclerosis per se? *Osteoporosis International* 18(4):505-512.

Balasubramanyam, M., A. A. Koteswari, R. S. Kumar, S. F. Monickaraj, J. U. Maheswari, and V. Mohan. 2003. Curcumin-induced inhibition of cellular reactive oxygen species generation: Novel therapeutic implications. *Journal of Biosciences* 28(6):715-721.

Barker, M. E., E. McCloskey, S. Saha, F. Gossiel, D. Charlesworth, H. J. Powers, et al. 2005. Serum retinoids and ß-carotene as predictors of hip and other fractures in elderly women. *Journal of Bone and Mineral Research* 20(6):913-920.

Bengmark, S. 2006. Curcumin, an atoxic antioxidant and natural NFκB, cyclooxygenase-2, lipooxygenase, and inducible nitric oxide synthase inhibitor: A shield against acute and chronic diseases. *American Society for Parenteral and Enteral Nutrition* 30(1):45-51.

Bessinger, J., and T. Yablon-Brenner. 2009. *Simple Food for Busy Families: The Whole Life Nutrition Approach.* Berkeley, CA: Ten Speed Press.

Bikle, D. D. 2007. Vitamin insufficiency/deficiency in gastrointestinal disorder. *Journal of Bone and Mineral Research* 22(Suppl 2):V50-V54.

Blanuša, M., V. Varnai, V. M. Piasek, and K. Kostial. 2005. Chelators as antidotes of metal toxicity: Therapeutic and experimental aspects. *Current Medicinal Chemistry* 12(23):2771-2794.

Bolland, M. J., P. A. Barber, R. N. Doughty, B. Mason, A. Horne, R. Ames, et al. 2008. Vascular events in healthy older women receiving calcium supplementation: Randomised controlled trial. *British Medical Journal* 336 (7638):262-266.

Brandao-Burch, A. 2003. Mild acidosis upregulates mRNA for cathepsin K and Traf-6, increases OC activity, and decreases OB function. 30th European Symposium on Calcified Tissues. Rome, Italy, May 8-12.

Brzóska, M. M., and J. Moniuszko-Jakoniuk. 2004. Low-level exposure to cadmium during the lifetime increases the risk of osteoporosis and fractures of the lumbar spine in the elderly: Studies on a rat model of human environmental exposure. *Toxicological Sciences* 82(2):468-477.

Bügel, S. 2003. Vitamin K and bone health. *Proceedings of the Nutrition Society* 62(4):839-843.

Caldwell, J. D., F. Suleman, S. H. H. Chou, R. Shapiro, Z. Herbert, and G. F. Jirikowski. 2006. Emerging roles of steroid-binding globulins. *Hormone and Metabolic Research* 38: 206-218.

Campbell, J. R., and P. Auinger. 2007. The association between blood lead levels and osteoporosis among adults—Results from the Third National Health and Nutrition Examination Survey (NHANES III). *Environmental Health Perspectives* 115(7):1018-1022.

Cao, J. J., P. Kurimoto, B. Boudignon, C. Rosen, F. Lima, and B. P. Halloran. 2007. Aging impairs IGF-1 receptor activation and induces skeletal resistance to IGF-1. *Journal of Bone and Mineral Research* 22(8):1271-1279.

Carmouche, J. J., J. E. Puzas, X. Zhang, P. Tiyapatanaputi, D. A. Cory-Slechta, R. Gelein, et al. 2005. Lead exposure inhibits fracture healing and is associated with increased chondrogenesis, delay in cartilage mineralization, and a decrease in osteoprogenitor frequency. *Environmental Health Perspectives* 113(6):749-755.

Cauley, J. A., S. R. Cummings, D. G. Seeley, D. Black, W. Browner, L. H. Kuller, et al. 1993. Effects of thiazide diuretic therapy on bone mass, fractures, and falls. The Study of Osteoporotic Fractures Research Group. *Annals of Internal Medicine* 118(9):666-673.

Cauley, J. A., M. E. Danielson, R. M. Boudreau, K. Y. Z. Forrest, J. M. Zmuda, M. Pahor, et al. 2007. Inflammatory markers and incident fracture risk in older men and women: The health aging and body composition study. *Journal of Bone and Mineral Research* 22(7):1088-1095.

Cauley, J. A., L. M. Salamone, and F. L. Lucas. 1996. Postmenopausal endogenous and exogenous hormones, degree of obesity, thiazide diuretics, and risk of osteoporosis. In *Osteoporosis,* edited by R. Marcus, D. Feldman, and J. Kelsey. San Diego, CA: Academic Press.

Cerf-Bensussan, N., T. Matysiak-Budnik, C. Cellier, and M. Heyman. 2007. Oral proteases: A new approach to managing coeliac disease. *Gut* 56(2):157-160.

Chesnut, C. H., III, M. Azria, S. Silverman, M. Engelhardt, M. Olsen, and L. Mindeholm. 2008. Salmon calcitonin: A review of current and future therapeutic indications. *Osteoporosis International* 19(4):479-491.

Chesnut, C. H., III, S. Majumdar, D. C. Newitt, A. Shields, J. van Pelt, E. Laschansky, et al. 2005. Effects of salmon calcitonin on trabecular microarchitecture as determined by magnetic resonance imaging: Results from the QUEST study. *Journal of Bone and Mineral Research* 20(9):1548-1561.

Chesnut, C. H. III, S. Silverman, K. Andriano, H. Genant, A. Gimona, S. Harris, et al. 2000. A randomized trial of nasal spray salmon calcitonin in postmenopausal women with established osteoporosis: The Prevent Recurrence of Osteoporosis Fractures Study. *American Journal of Medicine* 109(4):267-276.

Chrischilles, E. A., C. D. Butler, C. S. Davis, and R. B. Wallace. 1991. A model of lifetime osteoporosis impact. *Archives of Internal Medicine* 151(10):2026-2032.

Cornich, J., K. E. Callon, and I. R. Reid. 1996. Insulin increases histomorphometric indices of bone formation in vivo. *Calcified Tissue International* 59(6):492-495.

Costedio, M. M., N. Hyman, and G. M. Mawe. 2007. Serotonin and its role in colonic function and in gastrointestinal disorders. *Diseases of the Colon and Rectum* 50(3):376-388.

Cummings, S. R., S. Eckert, K. A. Krueger, D. Grady, T. J. Powles, J. A. Cauley, et al. 1999. The effect of raloxifene on risk of breast cancer in postmenopausal women. *Journal of the American Medical Association* 281(23):2189-2197.

de Vries, F., A. L. Cooper, R. F. Logan, S. M. Cockle, T. P. van Staa, and C. Cooper. 2008. Risk of fracture in postmenopausal women taking concomitant bisphosphonate and acid-suppressant medication. *Osteoporosis International* 19(Suppl 1):S20.

Deyhim, F., M. Kranthi, G. K. Jayaprakasha, and B. S. Patil. 2006. Grapefruit juice influences bone quality in orchidectomized and non-orchidectomized male rats. *Journal of Bone and Mineral Research* (Abstracts) 21(Suppl 1):S419.

Ding, C., V. Parameswaran, R. Udayan, J. Burgess, and G. Jones. 2008. Circulating levels of inflammatory markers predict change in bone mineral density and resorption in older adults: A longitudinal study. *Journal of Clinical Endocrinology and Metabolism* 93(5):1952-1958.

Dong, W., P. P. Simeonova, R. Gallucci, J. Matheson, L. Flood, S. Wang, et al. 1998. Toxic metals stimulate inflammatory cytokines in hepatocytes through oxidative stress mechanisms. *Toxicology and Applied Pharmacology* 151(2):359-366.

Eastell, R., J. H. Krege, P. Chen, E. V. Glass, and J. Y. Reginster. 2006. Development of an algorithm for using P1NP to monitor treatment of patients with teriparatide. *Current Medical Research and Opinion* 22(1):61-66.

Effenberger, K. E., S. A. Johnsen, D. G. Monroe, T. C. Spelsberg, and J. J. Westendorf. 2005. Regulation of osteoblastic phenotype and gene expression by hop-derived phytoestrogens. *Journal of Steroid Biochemistry and Molecular Biology* 96(5):387-399.

Elshafie, M. A. A., and A. A. A. Ewies. 2007. Transdermal natural progesterone cream for postmenopausal women: Inconsistent data and complex pharmacokinetics. *Journal of Obstetrics and Gynaecology* 27(7):655-659.

Ershler, W. B. 2003. Biological interactions of aging and anemia: A focus on cytokines. *Journal of the American Geriatrics Society* 51(Suppl 3):S18-S21.

Ettinger B., K. E. Ensrud, R. Wallace, K. C. Johnson, S. R. Cummings, V. Yankov, et al. 2004. Effects of ultralow-dose transdermal estradiol on bone mineral density: A randomized clinical trial. *Obstetrics and Gynecology* 104(3):443-451.

Farhat, G. N., A. B. Newman, K. Sutton-Tyrrell, K. A. Matthews, R. Boudreau, A. V. Schwartz, et al. 2007. The association of bone mineral density measures with incident cardiovascular disease in older adults. *Osteoporosis International* 18(7):999-1008.

Farooki, A., M. Fornnier, and C. Estilo. 2008. Retrospective analysis of biochemical markers of bone turnover in oncologic patients who developed osteonecrosis of the jaw. *Clinical and Experimental Metastasis* 25(Suppl 1):S53.

Feskanich D., V. Singh, W. C. Willett, and G. A. Colditz. 2002. Vitamin A intake and hip fractures among postmenopausal women. *Journal of the American Medical Association* 287(1):47-54.

Figura, N., L. Gennari, D. Merlotti, C. Lenzi, S. Campagna, B. Franci, et al. 2005. Prevalence of *Helicobacter pylori* infection in male patients with osteoporosis and controls. *Digestive Diseases and Sciences* 50(5):847-852.

Fitzgerald, K. N., C. Nelson-Dooley, and R. S. Lord. 2008. Nutrient and toxic elements. In *Laboratory Evaluations for Integrative and Functional Medicine*, 2nd ed., edited by R. S. Lord and J. A. Bralley. Duluth, GA: Metametrix Institute.

Frings-Meuthen, P., N. Baecker, and M. Heer. 2008. Low-grade metabolic acidosis may be the cause of sodium chloride-induced exaggerated bone resorption. *Journal of Bone and Mineral Research* 23(4):517-524.

Ganesan, K, S. Teklehaimanot, T. H. Tran, M. Asuncion, and K. Norris. 2005. Relationship of C-reactive protein and bone mineral density in community-dwelling elderly females. *Journal of the National Medical Association* 97(3):329-333.

Garnero, P., E. Hausherr, M. C. Chapuy, C. Marcelli, H. Grandjean, C. Muller, et al. 1996. Markers of bone resorption predict hip fracture in elderly women: The EPIDOS Prospective Study. *Journal of Bone and Mineral Research* 11(10):1531-1538.

Genant, H. K., K. Engelke, T. Fuerst, C. C. Glüer, S. Grampp, S. T. Harris, et al. 1996. Noninvasive assessment of bone mineral and structure: State of the art. *Journal of Bone and Mineral Research* 11(6):707-730.

Genuis, S. J., and G. K. Schwalfenberg. 2007. Picking a bone with contemporary osteoporosis management: Nutrient strategies to enhance skeletal integrity. *Clinical Nutrition* 26(2):193-207.

Gjesdal, C. G., S. E. Vollset, P. M. Ueland, H. Refsum, H. E. Meyer, and G. S. Tell. 2007. Plasma homocysteine, folate and vitamin B_{12} and the risk of hip fracture: The Hordaland Homocysteine Study. *Journal of Bone and Mineral Research* 22(5):747-756.

Gordon, C. M., E. Grace, S. J. Emans, H. A. Feldman, E. Goodman, K. A. Becker, et al. 2002. Effects of oral dehydroepiandrosterone on bone density in young women with anorexia nervosa: A randomized trial. *Journal of Clinical Endocrinology and Metabolism* 87(11):4935-4941.

Gordon, C. M., E. Grace, S. J. Emans, E. Goodman, M. H. Crawford, and M. S. Leboff. 1999. Changes in bone turnover markers and menstrual function after short-term oral DHEA in young women with anorexia nervosa. *Journal of Bone and Mineral Research* 14(1):136-145.

Grassi, F., M. Robbie-Ryan, W. Qian, K. Page, and R. Pacifici. 2005. Oxidative stress induced dendritic cell-dependent T cell activation: A novel mechanism by which estrogen deficiency causes bone loss. *Journal of Bone and Mineral Research* (Abstracts) 20(Suppl 1):S37.

Grassi, F., G. Tell, M. Robbie-Ryan, Y. Gao, M. Terauchi, X. Yang, et al. 2007. Oxidative stress causes bone loss in estrogen-deficient mice through enhanced bone marrow dendritic cell activation. *Proceedings of the National Academy of Sciences* 104(38):15087-15092.

Greenspan, S. L., and M. M. Luckey. 2006. Evaluation of postmenopausal osteoporosis. In *Primer on the Metabolic Bone Diseases and Disorders of Mineral Metabolism*, 6th ed., edited by M. J. Favus. Washington, DC: American Society for Bone and Mineral Research.

Hall, A. J., J. G. Babish, G. K. Darland, B. J. Carroll, V. R. Konda, R. H. Lerman, et al. 2008. Safety, efficacy and anti-inflammatory activity of rho iso-alpha-acids from hops. *Phytochemistry* 69(7):1534-1547.

He, F. J., N. D. Markandu, R. Coltart, J. Barron, and G. A. MacGregor. 2005. Effects of short-term supplementation of potassium chloride and potassium citrate on blood pressure in hypertensives. *Hypertension* 45(4):571-574.

Heaney, R. P. 2003. Quantifying human calcium absorption using pharmacokinetic methods. *Journal of Nutrition* 133(4):1224-1226.

Heaney, R. P., R. Carey, and L. Harkness. 2005. Roles of vitamin D, n-3 polyunsaturated fatty acid, and soy isoflavones in bone health. *Journal of the American Dietetic Association* 105(11):1700-1702.

Heffernan, M. P., K. G. Saag, J. K. Robinson, and J. P. Callen. 2006. Prevention of osteoporosis associated with chronic glucocorticoid therapy. *Journal of the American Medical Association* 295(11):1300-1303.

Helms, S. 2005. Celic disease and gluten-associated diseases. *Alternative Medicine Review* 10(3):172-192.

Hofbauer, L. C., C. C. Brueck, C. M. Shanahan, M. Schoppet, and H. Dobnig. 2007. Vascular calcification and osteoporosis: From clinical observation towards molecular understanding. *Osteoporosis International* 18(3):251-259.

Holick, M. F., E. S. Siris, N. Binkley, M. K. Beard, A. Khan, J. T. Katzer, et al. 2005. Prevalence of vitamin D inadequacy among postmenopausal North American women receiving osteoporosis therapy. *Journal of Clinical Endocrinology and Metabolism* 90(6):3215-3224.

Holloway, W. R., F. M. Collier, C. J. Aitken, D. E. Myers, J. M. Hodge, M. Malakellis, et al. 2002. Leptin inhibits osteoclast generation. *Journal of Bone and Mineral Research* 17(2):200-209.

Hsu, Y. L., and P. L. Kuo. 2008. Diosmetin induces human osteoblastic differentiation through the protein kinase C/p38 and extracellular signal-regulated kinase ½ pathway. *Journal of Bone and Mineral Research* 23(6):949-960.

Hu, J. P., K. Nishishita, E. Sakai, H. Yoshida, Y. Kato, T. Tsukuba, et al. 2008. Berberine inhibits RANKL-induced osteoclast formation and survival through suppressing the NF-kappaB and Akt pathways. *European Journal of Pharmacology* 580(1-2):70-79.

Huang, C., Y. Zhang, Z. Gong, X. Sheng, Z. Li, W. Zhang, et al. 2006. Berberine inhibits 3T3-L1 adipocyte differentiation through the PPAR gamma pathway. *Biochemical and Biophysical Research Communications* 348(2):571-578.

James, S. P. 2005. National Institutes of Health Consensus Development Conference Statement on Celiac Disease, June 28-30, 2004. *Gastroenterology* 128(4)(Suppl 1):S1-S9.

Jandziszak, K., C. Suarez, E. Wasserman, R. Clark, B. Baker, F. Liu, et al. 1998. Disturbances of growth hormone-insulin-like growth factor axis and response to growth hormone in acidosis. *American Journal of Physiology* 275(1, pt 2):R120-R128.

Järup, L. 2002. Cadmium overload and toxicity. *Nephrology, Dialysis, Transplantation* 17(Suppl 2):35-39.

Järup, L., and T. Alfvén. 2004. Low level cadmium exposure, renal and bone effects: The OSCAR study. *Biometals* 17(5):505-509.

Jehle, S., A. Zanetti, J. Muser, H. N. Hulter, and R. Krapf. 2005. Neutralization of the acidogenic Western diet with K citrate increases DXA BMD in postmenopausal (PM) osteopenic women: Results of a DBRCT. *Journal of Bone and Mineral Research* (Abstracts) 20(1):S289.

Jellin, J. M., P. J. Gregory, F. Batz, K. Hitchens, et al. 2006. Pharmacist's Letter/Prescriber's Letter. Natural Medicines Comprehensive Database, 8th ed. Stockton, CA: Therapeutic Research Facility.

Jones, D. S., and S. Quinn, eds. 2006. *Textbook of Functional Medicine.* Gig Harbor, WA: The Institute for Functional Medicine.

Jordan, J. 2005. Good vibrations and strong bones? *American Journal of Physiology. Regulatory, Integrative and Comparative Physiology* 288(3):R555-R556.

Jurutka, P. W., L. Bartik, G. K. Whitfield, D. R. Mathern, T. K. Barthel, M. Gurevich, et al. 2007 Vitamin D receptor: Key roles in bone mineral pathophysiology, molecular mechanism of action, and novel nutritional ligands. *Journal of Bone and Mineral Research* 22(Suppl 2):V2-V10.

Kahn, A. J., and B. Halloran. 2002. Dehydroepiandrosterone supplementation and bone turnover in middle-aged to elderly men. *Journal of Clinical Endocrinology and Metabolism* 87(4):1544-1549.

Kanis, J. A., O. Johnell, A. Oden, H. Johansson, and E. McCloskey. 2008. FRAX™ and the assessment of fracture probability in men and women from the UK. *Osteoporosis International* 19(4):385-397.

Kawada, E., K. Moridaira, K. Itoh, A. Hoshino, J. Tamura, and T. Morita. 2006. In long-term bedridden elderly patients with dietary copper deficiency, biochemical markers of bone resorption are increased with copper supplementation during 12 weeks. *Annals of Nutrition and Metabolism.* 50(5):420-424.

Khalil, N., J. A. Cauley, J. W. Wilson, E. O. Talbott, L. Morrow, M. C. Hochberg, et al. 2008. Relationship of blood lead levels in incident non-spine fractures and falls in older women: The Study of Osteoporotic Fractures. *Journal of Bone and Mineral Research* 23(9):1417-1425.

Knapen, M. H. J., L. J. Schurgers, and C. Vermeer. 2007. Vitamin K_2 supplementation improves hip bone geometry and bone strength indicies in postmenopausal women. *Osteoporosis International* 18(7):963-972.

Kramm, H. L., and K. E. Hansen. 2006. Hypovitaminosis D is common in physicians but measurement does not affect patient care. *Journal of Clinical Densitometry* 9(2):242.

Kress, B. C., I. A. Mizrahi, K. W. Armour, R. Marcus, R. D. Emkey, and A. C. Santora, II. 1999. Use of bone alkaline phosphatase to monitor alendronate therapy in individual postmenopausal osteoporotic women. *Clinical Chemistry* 45(7):1009-1017.

Lauretani, F., R. D. Semba, S. Bandinelli, A. L. Ray, J. M. Guralnik, and L. Ferrucci. 2007. Association of low plasma selenium concentrations with poor muscle strength in older community-dwelling adults: The InCHIANTI Study. *American Journal of Clinical Nutrition* 86(2):347-352.

Lean, J. M., J. T. Davies, K. Fuller, C. J. Jagger, B. Kirstein, G. A. Partington, et al. 2003. A crucial role for thiol antioxidants in estrogen-deficiency bone loss. *Journal of Clinical Investigation* 112(6):915-923.

Lee, D. H., I. K. Lee, M. Steffes, and D. R. Jacobs, Jr. 2007. Extended analysis of the association between serum concentrations of persistent organic pollutants and diabetes. *Diabetes Care* 30(6):1596-1598.

Lee, H. W., J. H. Suh, H. N. Kim, A. Y. Kim, S. Y. Park, C. S. Shin, et al. 2008. Berberine promotes osteoblast differentiation by Runx2 activation with p38 MAPK. *Journal of Bone and Mineral Research* 23(8):1227-1237.

Lee, N. K., H. Sowa, E. Hinoi, M. Ferron, J. D. Ahn, C. Confravreux, et al. 2007. Endocrine regulation of energy metabolism by the skeleton. *Cell* 130(3):456-469.

Leelawattana R., K. Ziambaras, J. Roodman-Weiss, C. Lyss, D. Wagner, T. Klug, et al. 2000. The oxidative metabolism of estradiol conditions postmenopausal bone density and bone loss. *Journal of Bone and Mineral Research* 15(12):2513-2520.

Lewiecki, E. M., J. P. Bilezikian, C. Cooper, M. C. Hochberg, M. M. Luckey, M. Maricic, et al. 2008. Proceedings of the Eighth Annual Santa Fe Bone Symposium, August 3-4, 2007. *Journal of Clinical Densitometry* 11(2):313-324.

Li, H., T. Miyahara, Y. Tezuka, Q. L. Tran, H. Seto, and S. Kadota. 2003. Effect of berberine on bone mineral density in SAMP6 as a senile osteoporosis model. *Biological and Pharmaceutical Bulletin* 26(1):110-111.

Lindsay, R., J. C. Gallagher, M. Kleerekoper, and J. H. Pickar. 2002. Effect of lower doses of conjugated equine estrogens with and without medroxyprogesterone acetate on bone in early postmenopausal women. *Journal of the American Medical Association* 287(20):2668-2676.

Liu, G., P. Men, G. H. Kenner, and S. C. Miller. 2008. Therapeutic effects of an oral chelator targeting skeletal tissue damage in experimental postmenopausal osteoporosis in rats. *Hemoglobin* 32(1-2):181-190.

Lord, R. S., and J. A. Bralley, eds. 2008. *Laboratory Evaluations for Integrative and Functional Medicine,* 2nd ed. Duluth, GA: Metametrix Institute.

Lowe, N. M., W. D. Fraser, and M. J. Jackson. 2002. Is there a potential therapeutic value of copper and zinc for osteoporosis? *Proceedings of the Nutrition Society* 61(2):181-185.

Lukaczer, D. 2006. The "4R" program. In *Textbook of Functional Medicine,* edited by D. S. Jones and S. Quinn. Gig Harbor, WA: The Institute for Functional Medicine.

Lyritis, G. P., N. Tsakalakos, B. Magiasis, T. Karachalios, A. Yiatzides, and M. Tsekoura. 1991. Analgesic effect of salmon calcitonin in osteoporotic vertebral fractures: A double-blind placebo-controlled clinical study. *Calcified Tissue International* 49(6):369-372.

Maggio, D., M. Barabani, M. Pierandrei, M. C. Polidori, M. Catani, P. Mecocci, et al. 2003. Marked decrease in plasma antioxidants in aged osteoporotic women: Results of a cross-sectional study. *Journal of Clinical Endocrinology and Metabolism* 88(4):1523-1527.

Maggio, M., S. Basaria, A. Ble, F. Lauretani, S. Bandinelli, G. P. Ceda, et al. 2006. Correlation between testosterone and the inflammatory marker soluble interleukin-6 receptor in older men. *Journal of Clinical Endocrinology and Metabolism* 91(1):345-347.

Malluche, H. H. 2002. Aluminum and bone disease in chronic renal failure. *Nephrology, Dialysis, Transplantation* 17(suppl 2):21-24.

Marie, P. J., M. T. Garba, M. Hott, and L. Miravet. 1985. Effect of low doses of stable strontium on bone metabolism in rats. *Mineral and Electrolyte Metabolism* 11(1):5-13.

Martino, S., J. A. Cauley, E. Barrett-Connor, T. J. Powles, J. Mershon, D. Disch, et al. 2004. Continuing outcomes relevant to Evista: Breast cancer incidence in postmenopausal osteoporotic women in a randomized trial of raloxifene. *Journal of the National Cancer Institute* 96(23):1751-1761.

Mathey, J., J. Mardon, N. Fokialakis, C. Puel, S. Kati-Coulibaly, S. Mitakou, et al. 2007. Modulation of soy isoflavones bioavailability and subsequent effects on bone health in ovariectomized rats: The case for equol. *Osteoporosis International* 18(5):671-679.

Mattila, P., M. Svanberg, and M. Knuuttila. 2001. Increasing bone volume and bone mineral content in Xylitol-fed aged rats. *Gerontology* 47(6):300-305.

Matysiak-Budnik, T., I. C. Moura, M. Arcos-Fajardo, C. Lebreton, S. Ménard, C. Candalh, et al. 2008. Secretory IgA mediates retrotranscytosis of intact gliadin peptides via the transferring receptor in celiac disease. *The Journal of Experimental Medicine* 205(1): 143-154.

McLean, R. R., P. F. Jacques, J. Selhub, K. L. Tucker, E. J. Samelson, K. E. Broe, et al. 2004. Homocysteine as a predictive factor for hip fracture in older persons. *New England Journal of Medicine* 350(20):2042-2049.

Melkko, J., S. Kauppila, S. Niemi, L. Risteli, K. Haukipuro, A. Jukkola, et al. 1996. Immunoassay for intact amino-terminal propeptide of human type 1 procollagen. *Clinical Chemistry* 42(6):947-954.

Meunier, P. J., C. Roux, E. Seeman, S. Ortolani, J. E. Badurski, T. D. Spector, et al. 2004. The effects of strontium ranelate on the risk of vertebral fractures in postmenopausal women with osteoporosis. *New England Journal of Medicine* 350(5):459-468.

Miekeley, N., L. M. de Carvalho Fortes, C. L. Porto da Silveira, and M. B. Lima. 2001. Elemental anomalies in hair as indicators of endocrinologic pathologies and deficiencies in calcium and bone metabolism. *Journal of Trace Elements in Medicine and Biology* 15(1):46-55.

Morabito, N., A. Crisafulli, C. Vergara, A. Gaudio, A. Lasco, N. Frisina, et al. 2003. Effects of genistein and hormone-replacement therapy on bone loss in early postmenopausal women: A randomized double-blind placebo-controlled study. *Journal of Bone and Mineral Research* 17(10):1904-1912.

Nagata, M., A. Suzuki, S. Sekiguchi, Y. Ono, K. Nishiwaki-Yasuda, T. Itoi, et al. 2007. Subclinical hypothyroidism is related to lower heel QUS in postmenopausal women. *Endocrine Journal* 54(4):625-630.

Nash, D., L. S. Magder, R. Sherwin, R. J. Rubin, and E. K. Silbergeld. 2004. Bone density-related predictors of blood lead level among peri- and post-menopausal women in the United States. *American Journal of Epidemiology* 160(9):901-911.

National Osteoporosis Foundation. 2008. *Clinician's Guide to Prevention and Treatment of Osteoporosis.* Washington, DC: National Osteoporosis Foundation.

Need, A. G., M. Horowitz, H. A. Morris, R. Moore, and C. Nordin. 2007. Seasonal change in osteoid thickness and mineralization lag time in ambulant patients. *Journal of Bone and Mineral Research* 22(5):757-761.

Neviaser, A. S., J. M. Lane, B. A. Lenart, F. Edobor-Osula, and D. G. Lorich. 2008. Low-energy femoral shaft fractures associated with alendronate use. *Journal of Orthopaedic Trauma* 22(5):346-350.

Nugmanova, L. B., A. Y. Kandilyotu, K. Y. Agababyan, and V. M. Vorojeikin. 2006. Comparison of the treatment effect of ossein-hydroxyapatite compound and calcium carbonate with vitamin D_3 on bone tissue histomorphometric parameters in the ovariectomized (OVX) rats. *Osteoporosis International* 17(Suppl 1):S23.

Obermayer-Pietsch, B. M., M. Gugatschka, S. Reitter, W. Plank, A. Strele, D. Walter, et al. 2007. Adult-type hypolactasia and calcium availability: Decreased calcium intake or impaired calcium absorption? *Osteoporosis International* 18(4):445-451.

Ohlsson, C., L. Vandenput, A. Holmberg, H. Mallmin, E. Orwoll, A. Oden, et al. 2007. Serum DHEA is independently of estradiol and testosterone related to incident fractures in elderly men—the MrOS Sweden Study. *Journal of Bone and Mineral Research* (Abstracts) 22(Suppl 1):S56.

Palacios, C. 2006. The role of nutrients in bone health, from A to Z. *Critical Reviews in Food Science and Nutrition* 46(8):621-628.

Parhami, F. 2003. Possible role of oxidized lipids in osteoporosis: Could hyperlipidemia be a risk factor? *Prostaglandins, Leukotrienes, and Essential Fatty Acids* 68(6):373-378.

Parhami, F., B. Basseri, J. Hwang, Y. Tintut, and L. L. Demer. 2002. High-density lipoprotein regulates calcification of vascular cells. *Circulation Research* 91(7):570-576.

Park, H., A. Yasunaga, E. Watanabe, F. Togo, S. Park, K. Yoshiuchi, et al. 2007. Interactive effects of milk basic protein supplementation and habitual physical activity on bone health in older women: A 1-year randomized controlled trial from the Nakanojo Study. *Journal of Bone and Mineral Research* (Abstracts) 22(Suppl 1):S448.

Pasco, J. A., M. A. Kotowicz, M. J. Henry, G. C. Nicholson, H. J. Spilsbury, J. D. Box, et al. 2006. High-sensitivity C-reactive protein and fracture risk in elderly women. *Journal of the American Medical Association* 296(11):1353-1355.

Paterson, B. M., K. M. Lammers, M. C. Arrieta, A. Fasano, and J. B. Meddings. 2007. The safety, tolerance, pharmacokinetic and pharmacodynamic effects of single doses of AT-1001 in celiac disease subjects: A proof of concept study. *Alimentary Pharmacology and Therapeutics* 26(5):757-766.

Patrick, L. 2002. Mercury toxicity and antioxidants: Part 1. Role of glutathione and alpha-lipoic acid in the treatment of mercury toxicity. *Alternative Medicine Review* 7(6):456-471.

Pizzorno, J. E., Jr., and M. T. Murray, eds. 2000. *Textbook of Natural Medicine*, 2nd ed. London: Harcourt Publishers Limited.

Pogoda, P., M. Egermann, J. C. Schnell, M. Priemel, A. F. Schilling, M. Alini, et al. 2006. Leptin inhibits bone formation not only in rodents, but also in sheep. *Journal of Bone and Mineral Research* 21(10):1591-1599.

Pogrel, M. A. 2004. Bisphosphonates and bone necrosis. *Journal of Oral and Maxillofacial Surgery* 62(3):391-392.

Prince, R. L., A. Devine, S. S. Dhaliwal, and I. M. Dick. 2004. Results of 5 year double-blind, placebo-controlled trial of calcium supplementation (CAIFOS): Clinical fracture outcomes. *Journal of Bone and Mineral Research* (Abstracts) 19(Suppl 1):S3.

Prouillet, C., J. C. Mazière, C. Mazière, A. Wattel, M. Brazier, and S. Kamel. 2004. Stimulatory effect of naturally occurring flavonols quercetin and kaempferol on alkaline phosphatase activity in MG-63 human osteoblasts through ERK and estrogen receptor pathway. *Biochemical Pharmacology* 67(7):1307-1313.

Quan, Z. F., C. Yang, N. Li, and J. S. Li. 2004. Effects of glutamine on change in early postoperative intestinal permeability and its relation to systemic inflammation response in early postoperative patients. *Gastroenterology* 10(13):1992-1994.

Quig, D. 1998. Cysteine metabolism and metal toxicity. *Alternative Medicine Review* 3(4):262-270.

Rao, L. G., E. S. MacKinnon, R. G. Josse, T. M. Murray, A. Strauss, and A. V. Rao. 2007. Lycopene consumption decreases oxidative stress and bone resorption markers in postmenopausal women. *Osteoporosis International* 18(1):109-115.

Reid, I. R. 2002. Relationships among body mass, its components, and bone. *Bone* 31(5):547-555.

Reid, I. R., J. Cornish, and P. A. Baldock. 2006. Perspective: Nutrition-related peptides and bone homeostasis. *Journal of Bone and Mineral Research* 21(4):495-500.

Revilla, M., L. F. Villa, A. Sanchez-Atrio, and R. H. Hernandez. 1997. Influence of body mass index on the age-related slope of total and regional bone mineral content. *Calcified Tissue International* 61(2):134-138.

Riggs, B. L., and L. J. Melton III. 1995. The worldwide problem of osteoporosis: Insights afforded by epidemiology. *Bone* 17(5 Suppl):505S-511S.

Rosen, C. J., C. Ackert-Bicknell, W. G. Beamer, T. Nelson, M. Adamo, P. Cohen, et al. 2005. Allelic differences in a quantitative trait locus affecting insulin-like growth factor-I impact skeleton acquisition and body composition. *Pediatric Nephrology* 20(3):255-260.

Rosen, C. J., and M. L. Bouxsein. 2006. Mechanisms of disease: Is osteoporosis the obesity of bone? *Nature Clinical Practice. Rheumatology* 2(1):35-43.

Rubin, C., R. Recker, D. Cullen, J. Ryaby, J. McCabe, and K. McLeod. 2004. Prevention of postmenopausal bone loss by a low-magnitude, high-frequency mechanical stimuli: A clinical trial assessing compliance, efficacy, and safety. *Journal of Bone and Mineral Research* 19(3):343-351.

Rubin, C., A. S. Turner, S. Bain, C. Mallinckrodt, and K. McLeod. 2001. Low mechanical signals strengthen long bones. *Nature* 412:603-604.

Ruggiero, S. L., B. Mehrotra, T. J. Rosenberg, and S. L. Engroff. 2004. Osteonecrosis of the jaws associated with the use of bisphosphonates: A review of 63 cases. *Journal of Oral and Maxillofacial Surgery* 62(5):527-534.

Ryan, E. P., J. D. Holz, M. Mulcahey, T. J. Sheu, T. A. Gasiewicz, and J. E. Puzas. 2007. Environmental toxicants may modulate osteoblast differentiation by a mechanism involving the aryl hydrocarbon receptor. *Journal of Bone and Mineral Research* 22(10):1571-1580.

Saito, M., K. Fujii, S. Soshi, and T. Tanaka. 2006. Reductions in degree of mineralization and enzymatic collagen cross-links and increases in glycation-induced pentosidine in the femoral neck cortex in cases of femoral neck fracture. *Osteoporosis International* 17(7):986-995.

Salminen, H. S., M. Sääf, H. Ringertz, and L. Strender. 2007. The role of IGF-1 and IGFBP-1 status and secondary hyperparathyroidism in relation to osteoporosis in elderly Swedish women. *Journal of Bone and Mineral Research* (Abstracts) 22(1):S170.

Sanchez-Hidalgo, M., Z. Lu, D. X. Tan, M. D. Maldonado, R. J. Reiter, and R. I. Gregerman. 2007. Melatonin inhibits fatty acid-induced triglyceride accumulation in ROS17/2.8 cells: Implications for osteoblast differentiation and osteoporosis. *American Journal of Physiology. Regulatory, Integrative and Comparative Physiology* 292(6):R2208-R2215.

Schousboe, J. T., J. A. Nyman, R. L. Kane, and K. E. Ensrud. 2005. Cost-effectiveness of alendronate therapy for osteopenic postmenopausal women. *Annals of Internal Medicine* 142(9):734-741.

Schürch, M. A., R. Rizzoli, D. Slosman, L. Vadas, P. Vergnaud, and J. P. Bonjour. 1998. Protein supplements increase serum insulin-like growth factor-I levels and attenuate proximal femur bone loss in patients with recent hip fracture: A randomized, double-blind, placebo-controlled trial. *Annals of Internal Medicine* 128(10):801-809.

Setchell, K. D. R., and E. Lydeking-Olsen. 2003. Dietary phytoestrogens and their effect on bone: Evidence from in vitro and in vivo, human observational, and dietary intervention studies. *American Journal of Clinical Nutrition* 78(3):593S-609S.

Shahnazari, M., N. A. Sharkey, G. J. Fosmire, and R. M. Leach. 2006. Effects of strontium on bone strength, density, volume, and microarchitecture in laying hens. *Journal of Bone and Mineral Research* 21(11):1696-1703.

Shiraki, M., Y. Shiraki, C. Aoki, and M. Miura. 2000. Vitamin K_2 (menatrenone) effectively prevents fractures and sustains lumbar bone mineral density in osteoporosis. *Journal of Bone and Mineral Research* 15:515-521.

Sierra, E. M., and E. Tiffany-Castiglioni. 1992. Effects of low-level lead exposure on hypothalamic hormones and serum progesterone levels in pregnant guinea pigs. *Toxicology* 72(1):89-97.

Silbergeld, E. K., J. Sauk, M. Somerman, A. Todd, F. McNeill, B. Fowler, et al. 1993. Lead in bone: Storage site, exposure source, and target organ. *Neurotoxicology* 14(2-3):225-236.

Simpson, E. R., M. Misso, K. N. Hewitt, R. A. Hill, W. C. Boon, M. E. Jones, et al. 2005. Estrogen—the good, the bad, and the unexpected. *Endocrine Reviews* 26(3):322-330.

Specker, B. L., T. Binkley, M. Vukovich, and T. Beare. 2007. Volumetric bone mineral density and bone size in sleep-deprived individuals. *Osteoporosis International* 18(1):93-99.

Stenson, W. F., R. Newberry, R. Lorenz, C. Baldus, and R. Civitelli. 2005. Increased prevalence of celiac disease and need for routine screening among patients with osteoporosis. *Archives of Internal Medicine* 165(4):393-399.

Stevens, J. F., C. L. Miranda, B. Frei, and D. R. Buhler. 2003. Inhibition of peroxynitrite-mediated LDL oxidation by prenylated flavonoids: The alpha symbol t, ß-unsaturated keto functionality of 2′-hydroxychalcones as novel antioxidant pharmacophore. *Chemical Research in Toxicology* 16(10):1277-1286.

Stevens, R. G., D. Y. Jones, M. S. Micozzi, and P. R. Taylor. 1988. Body iron stores and the risk of cancer. *New England Journal of Medicine* 319(16):1047-1052.

Stewart, J. C., D. Janicki-Deverts, M. F. Muldoon, and T. W. Kamarck. 2008. Depressive symptoms moderate the influence of hostility on serum interleukin-6 and C-reactive protein. *Psychosomatic Medicine* 70(2):197-204.

Takada, Y., S. Aoe, and M. Kumegawa. 1996. Whey protein stimulates the proliferation and differentiation of osteoblastic MC3T3-E1 cells. *Biochemical and Biophysical Research Communications* 223(2):445-449.

Takada, Y., N. Kobayashi, H. Matsuyama, K. Kato, J. Yamamura, M. Yahiro, et al. 1997. Whey protein suppresses the osteoclast-mediated bone resorption and osteoclast cell formation. *International Dairy Journal* 7(12):821-825.

Tankó, L. B., C. Christiansen, D. A. Cox, M. J. Geiger, M. A. McNabb, and S. R. Cummings. 2005. Relationship between osteoporosis and cardiovascular disease in postmenopausal women. *Journal of Bone and Mineral Research* 20(11):1912-1920.

Taranta, A., D. Fortunati, M. Longo, N. Rucci, E. Iacomino, F. Aliberti, et al. 2004. Imbalance of osteoclastogenesis-regulating factors in patients with celiac disease. *Journal of Bone and Mineral Research* 19(7):1112-1121.

Tobe, H., Y. Muraki, K. Kitamura, O. Komiyama, Y. Sato, T. Sugioka, et al. 1997. Bone resorption inhibitors from hop extract. *Bioscience, Biotechnology and Biochemistry* 61(1):158-159.

Travison, T. G., A. B. Araujo, G. R. Esche, and J. B. McKinlay. 2008. The relationship between body composition and bone mineral content: Threshold effects in a racially and ethnically diverse group of men. *Osteoporosis International* 19(1):29-38.

Van de Weijer, P. H. M., L. A. Mattsson, and O. Ylikorkala. 2007. Benefits and risks of long-term low-dose oral continuous combined hormone therapy. *Maturitas* 56(3):231-248.

Vermeer, C. 2004. Vitamin K and bone health. In *Nutritional Aspects of Osteoporosis,* 2nd ed., edited by P. Burckhardt, B. Dawson-Hughes, and R. P. Heaney. Burlington, MA: Elsevier Academic Press.

Wang, M. C., L. K. Bachrach, V. Loan, M. Hudes, K. M. Flegal, and P. B. Crawford. 2005. The relative contribution of lean tissue mass and fat mass to bone density in young women. *Bone* 37(4):474-481.

Warren, J. R., and B. Marshall. 1983. Unidentified curved bacilli on gastric epithelium in active chronic gastritis. *The Lancet* 1(8386):1273-1275.

Warren, M. P., and S. Halpert. 2004. Hormone replacement therapy: Controversies, pros and cons. *Best Practice and Research. Clinical Endocrinology and Metabolism* 18(3):317-332.

Werbach, M. R., and J. Moss. 1999. *Textbook of Nutritional Medicine.* Tarzana, CA.: Third Line Press.

Wittman, R., and H. Hu. 2002. Cadmium exposure and nephropathy in a 28-year-old female metals worker. *Environmental Health Perspectives* 110(2):1261-1266.

World Health Organization. 1994. Assessment of fracture risk and its application to screening for postmenopausal osteoporosis. WHO Technical Report Series 843. Geneva: World Health Organization.

Wu, J., J. Oka, I. Tabata, M. Higuchi, T. Toda, N. Fuku, et al. 2006. Effects of isoflavone and exercise on BMD and fat mass in postmenopausal Japanese women. *Journal of Bone and Mineral Research* 21(5):780-789.

Yadav, V. K., J. H. Ryu, N. Suda, K. F. Tanaka, J. A. Gingrich, G. Schütz, et al. 2008. Lrp5 controls bone formation by inhibiting serotonin synthesis in the duodenum. *Cell* 135:825-837.

Yamamura, J., S. Aoe, Y. Toba, M. Motouri, H. Kawakami, M. Kumegawa, et al. 2002. Milk basic protein (MBP) increases radial bone mineral density in healthy adult women. *Bioscience, Biotechnology, and Biochemistry* 66(3):702-704.

Yang, Y. X., J. D. Lewis, S. Epstein, and D. C. Metz. 2006. Long-term proton pump inhibitor therapy and risk of hip fracture. *Journal of the American Medical Association* 296(24):2947-2953.

R. Keith McCormick, DC, is a chiropractic physician in private practice in western Massachusetts specializing in the nutritional management of patients with bone fragility. McCormick studied human biology at Stanford University and earned his doctorate at the National College of Chiropractic. He is a member of the American Society for Bone and Mineral Research, the International Society of Clinical Densitometry, the American Chiropractic Association, and the Institute for Functional Medicine. McCormick is an Ironman triathlon competitor and a former U.S. Olympian (1976). Visit McCormick online at www.mccormickdc.com.

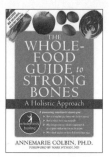
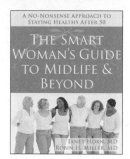
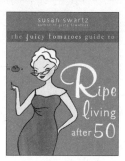
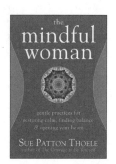
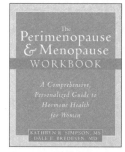
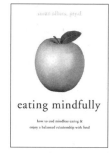